MĀNASOLLĀSA AND ĀYURVEDA

MĀNASOLLĀSA AND ĀYURVEDA

Mahadev N. Joshi
B.S. Hebbali

Foreword

Dr. N.P. Unni
Ex-Vice Chancellor
Sree Sankaracharya Sanskrit University
Kalady, Kerala

SHARADA

SHARADA PUBLISHING HOUSE
DELHI

First Published : 2004

ISBN : 81-85616-97-3

Published by :
B.L. Bansal
SHARADA PUBLISHING HOUSE
(Publishers on India's Past and Present)
40, Anand Nagar, Inder Lok,
Delhi-110035
Ph. : 23657538

Laser Typesetting by :
Creative Graphics
Ph. 22195643

Printed at :
Santosh Offset, Delhi-110035

FOREWORD

Sanskrit literature comprises all branches of learning, both general like Kāvya, Nāṭaka, Caṁpu, Alaṅkāra and Vṛtta and technical like the different Darsanas dealing with the six systems of Indian philosophy, Tantra, Śilpa, Vaidya, Gaṇita and Saṅgita. There are many patrons of literature who encouraged studies in these fields and some of them wrote several works pertaining to different fields. These fields are so vast and varied that historian have expressed the doubt that at least some of them were the contributions of their proteges. Works of encyclopaedic character are also prevalent in Sanskrit. Here again the author comprehends several fields of learning into the fold of his work. The finest example of this type is the Bṛhatsaṁhitā of Varāhamihira which contains one hundred chapters in addition to several appendices. It is said in the text :

शतग्विदमदयायानामनुपरिपाटिक्रमादनुक्रान्तम्।
अत्र श्लोकसहस्त्राण्याबद्धान्यूनचत्वारि।।

It has one hundred chapters and verses equivalent to 3900 ones of the ślokamatre. Some of the chapters have some relevance to medicine also.

चिह्नं गवामथ शुनां कुक्कटकूर्माजपुरुषचिह्नं च।
पञ्चमनुष्यविभागः स्त्रीचिह्न वस्त्रविच्छेदः।।

It treats of signs of cows, of dogs, of cocks, of tortoises, of goats, of horses and elephants, of men, of the five kinds of greatmen, of maidens and of seits of garments. In another chapter the characteristics of some of the above species are dealt with.

Tantrapaddhati also known as Iśānasiva gurudeva paddhati after its author Iśānasiva gurudeva is a significant work of encyclopaedia character in 118 paṭalās. Though the stress is on rituals the another has comprehended in his fold many subjects related to Āyurveda. This he has mentioned in his introductory verses as follows :

विस्तृतानि विशिष्टानि तन्त्राणि विविधान्यहम्।
यावत्सामनार्थमालोच्य करिष्ये तन्त्रपद्धतिम्।।

- - - - - - - - - - - - - - - - - - - -

विषग्रहामयादीनां प्रशमोपायदर्शिनीम्।
मन्त्रबिम्बौषधिध्यानैर्विद्यां सञ्जीवनीमिव।।
असुहृन्निग्रहोच्चाटविद्वेषस्तम्भमोहनैः।
उत्सादमारणोपायैर्दण्डनीतिमिवापराम्।।

Here the author compares his work of Sanjivanam, the divine elixir capable of restoring the dead to life since it contains the remedial measures for the affliction caused by poison, disease, evil magic etc. The following sections of the work are of great interest to a student of medicine,

केवलरोगशान्तिः गवाश्वादिशान्तिः, सर्पजातिभेदस्तदुत्पत्यादिक्रमश्च, दंशनभेदाः, तल्लक्षणानि, दष्टस्याबस्थाविशेषाश्च, फणिचिकित्सा, मण्डलिचिकित्सा, राजिलचिकित्सा, सर्वाद्रिचिकित्सा, वृश्चिकचिकित्सा, आखुविषचिकित्सा, लूताचिकित्सा, नानाप्राणिविषचिकित्सा, नानास्थावरद्रव्यविषचिकित्सा, खड्गरावण-बालचिकित्सा, बालपीडग्रहः, तत्प्रतीकारविधयश्च, ग्रहाणां भेदाः, अपस्मारोन्माद-चिकित्साधिकारः, गोरक्षाधिकारः, नानाद्रव्यभावनाधिकारः, आयुरियत्तावेदननिमित्तानि, आयुर्वर्धनरसायनविधि विशेषः, मृत्युविजयोपायः।

Thus it may be seen that the Tantrapaddhati deserves a careful study from the point of view of medicine. There are a few more such works on Tantra which incidentally deal with medicine. But some are of the view that the prescription contained in these works may be taken only as secondary sources. It is my firm view that without a comparison with original works on medicine these could not be considered as authoritative. Mānasollāsa itself has carved against quacks who practice medicine in the following works which are oft quoted in works on Subhāṣitas and Anthologies.

यमः क्रूरोभिषक् क्रूरो यमात्क्रूरतरोभिषक्।
यमस्तु हरतेप्राणान् वैद्यस्तु सवसूनसून्।।

वैद्यनाथ नमस्तुभ्यं मारिताशेषमानव
त्वयिविन्यस्तभारो यत् कृतान्तः सुखमेधते।।

It may be seen that the physician had an unenviable position in the society collecting bouquets and brickbats.

Someśvara's Mānasollāsa

Someśvaradeva of Cālukya dynasty has composed the Abhilaśitārthacintāmaṇi better and precisely known as Mānasollāsa. The first title is only an adjective to qualify the real name. In the work it is stated that–

The title is given at the end of the different chapters as 'Abhilaśitārthacintāmaṇi Rāja Mānasollāsa'. The editor of the original text R. Shama Sastry has noted as "Boon-stone of all desirable knowledge". He has observed that eventhough the title is suggestive of all branches of knowledge known at the time of the author, the subjects treated are very few. This incidentally includes enumeration of diseases, and their remedies. The scope is further enlarged by the details of training of horses and elephants together with the treatment of their diseases, preparation of liquor and beverages.

In the present monograph the elements dealing the Āyurveda are collected together for critical evaluation and treatment. The first chapter of the book deals with material according to Someśvara. The second chapter is an inquiry into the sources that may have been relied upon by Someśvara for which the statement- वैद्यशास्त्रानुसारेण कारयेत् तत् प्रतिक्रियां forms the basis for the author. Accordingly an account of ancient treatises on

Āyurveda is given here. Medical treatises of Caraka, Suśruta. Aṣṭāngasangraha and Aṣṭānga-hṛdaya of Vahata are the main works that are perused together with their mythological sources right from the times of Atharvaveda. The third chapter represents the concepts of Āyurveda. A list of 23 authors and their contributions to certain field of studies is given in this section. Naturally many of these are mentioned by Someśvara even though definite qualifications are wanting. The fourth chapter mentions the environmental aspects revealed by the texts in Āyurveda. The fifth and final chapter highlights the physical and mental health according to Someśvara's work. In the course of the treatment of the subject many factors relating to Āyurveda are provided for general information. The treatment of the subject of Āyurveda is made in connection with polity. The king should be careful against prisoning. Hence his cook has to be carefully watched in the preparation of food. For such matters the employment of physician is a must.

नराणां च गजानां च वाजिनां च गवामपि।।

मृगाणां च खगानां च ये जानन्ति चिकित्सितम्।।

परम्परागतास्सम्यगष्टाङ्गे तु चिकित्सिते।।

शस्त्रकर्मकलादक्षाः मन्त्रतन्त्रे च कोविदाः।
देहे च शीर्षिणफाले च विषे शल्ये ग्रहेऽपि च।।

वृष्ये रसायने चैव कुशला भिषजोऽष्टसु।
रोगनामनिदानं च रुजं जानान्ति तत्वतः।।

औषधं रूपनामभ्यां जानन्तो भिषजो वराः।
वमौ विरेचने नस्ये वस्तौ शस्त्रक्रियास्वापि।।

शस्यन्ते भिषजस्सम्यक् निष्णाताः पञ्चकर्मसु।
यत्किञ्चिदौषधैः साध्यं शरीरेषु हिताहितम्।।

सम्यग् विदन्ति ये वैद्या नृपयोग्या भवन्ति ते।
कृच्छ्र साध्यमसाध्यं वा जाड्यंजानन्ति तत्वतः।।

देशं कालं वायोऽवस्थां प्रकृतिं सात्म्यमेव च।
असाध्याः परक्रियाणां आत्मस्वामिहिते रताः।।
धर्मज्ञा दृढचित्ताश्च वैद्याः कार्या महीभुजा।।

In these lines the qualities of an ideal royal physician are noted by Someśvara. The physician should be proficient in the treatment of human beings, elephants, horses, cattle, animals, birds etc. He should know the traditional Aṣṭāngacikitsā and surgery in addition to being an expert in Mantrās and Tantrās. Diseases of the limbs, head, forehead, etc. should be treated. Expertise in toxicology (vesa), surgery (śalya), epilepsy (grahacikitsa), tonics (vrsya) and rasāyana (rejuvenation) is also expected of him. The names of the diseases, the basic principle of the ailments and the proper medicine for them should be understood by the Doctor/Physician. His ability to perform the traditional pancakarma like Vamana, Virecana, and Śastrakriyā must be tested before selection. He must also know whether the particular disease can be treated with oral application of medicine like decoction. Whether the treatment will be effective in a particular body is also to be investigated by the Physician. Place, time, age condition, nature and identity etc., should be kept in mind. He should be truthful and firm in matters regarding his own master. Such a physician alone should be selected by the king. Varāhamihira the author of Bṛhatsamhitā has well highlighted these aspects and Someśvara must have been influenced by this early treatise.

Secondary Literature

Shama Sastry has dealt with in his brief introduction subjects dealt with in the Mānasollāsa. It goes without saying that the book must be a compilation from different authoritative sources available to the king. For instance there are several works in Sanskrit dealing with elephantology like Palakapya, Rajadanta, Karnapura, Utpalamala, Matangalila etc., though most of them are known only at present through citation of commentators. The necessity for caring the elephants is made out as follows :

एकोविजयतेदन्ती मदघूर्णितलोचनः।
मुख्यं दन्तिबलं राज्ञां समरे विजयैषिणाम्।।

तस्मान्निजबले कार्या बहवो वारणोत्तमाः।
ततस्तेषां महीपालः पोषणे यत्नवान् भवेत्।।

Various diseases and their treatment relating to elephants are provided in this connection in manuals. In order to ascertain the exact source of one royal author one has to go through the originals. Similarly in dealing with horses, it is said :

साध्यन्ते तुरगैरेव दूरस्था अपि वैरिणः।
लभ्यते तुरगैः कीर्तिः यस्याश्वस्तस्य भूस्थिरा।।

The qualities of horses procured from different regions are enumerated. These are procured from various localities in India and abroad. Their ailments and remedial measures are also dealt with in this encyclopaedic work by Someśvara.

The present monograph highlights the importance of secondary sources of medicine since they contain much information hitherto not available in the standard treatises on Āyurveda. The attempts of the present authors Dr. M.N. Joshi and Dr. B.S. Hebbali deserves real praise from lovers of the Indian Systems of medicine which are now attracting international attention.

15, Nov. 2002
Trivandrum

Dr. N.P. Unni
Ex-Vice Chancellor
Sree Sankaracharya Sanskrit University
Kalady, Kerala

PREFACE

It gives me great pleasure to place before the circle of our Sanskrit readers, my book "Mānasollāsa and Āyurveda". In the present day life, which offers many temptations, we should not deviate from the path followed by our ancestors. Therefore, it is quite essential that we should gain proper knowledge from some of our ancient Treatises., That does help us to lead a peaceful and purposeful life on this earth.

I place on record my deep sense of gratitude to Dr. N.P. Unni, Ex-Vice-Chancellor, Sree Sankaracharya Sanskrit University, Kalady, Kerala for having graced this work 'Mānasollāsa and Āyurveda' with his valuable foreword and blessed me with best wishes from his heart of hearts. His valuable suggestions and guidelines have framed the soft corners of this work.

Many other scholars have encouraged and helped me in completing this work. Among them, mention has to be made of my teachers and colleagues. I express my gratitude to all these scholars for their help. I am grateful to my Ph. D. student Dr. B.S. Hebballi, Dept. of Sanskrit, BAMS College, Belgaum for his overall help in seeing this work through the press. My special thanks to Dr. V.B. Joshi, Dr. Subbray Bhat, Dr. Annapurna Hegde, Prof. S. Ramachandra, Dr. C.V. Venugopal and Prof. B.B. Hunagund for their help and encouragement.

My hearty thanks are also due to Creative Graphics, Delhi, for their pain taking, attention in bringing out this book so well.

Lastly, I also thank-Sharada Publishing House, Delhi for completing the printing in the quickest possible time. My efforts embolden me to seek good response from the readers.

Dharwad
21-11-2002

M.N. Joshi
Reader and Chairman,
Dept. of Sanskrit,
K. U., Dharwad

CONTENTS

1

MĀNASOLLĀSA AND ITS SIGNIFICANCE

Rāja Mānasollāsa popularly called Mānasollāsa is an encyclopaedic work of the western Cālukya King Someśvara III. It can be pointed out that this work was written by the author sparing most of his life-time to contribute richly to the world of knowledge. Rāja Mānasollāsa, also known as Abhilaṣitārth-acintāmaṇi, is a monumental work of the 12th century monarch, Someśvara III, of the Cālukya dynasty. He was a versatile person. He was an erudite Sanskrit scholar, a great warrior, an able administrator and a benevolent ruler of his subjects. In his renowned work, the ruler has outlined the duties and responsibilities of a king devoted to the well-being of his people.

Generally speaking, every person desires to achieve knowledge, brilliance of mind, wealth, strength and a robust health. In this respect, we are fortunate that our ancient sages and well-wishers have left their experiences and wisdom for our benefit. Many of these ancient concepts are still valid and are useful as guiding stars in our present day life. It is precisely for this reason that we have to study our ancient literature and the *Śāstras*.

The almost innate propensity of the ancient Indians, described above, gave birth to scientific treatises on different subjects. The ancients, for instance, wrote on दर्शन, व्याकरण, कोश, ज्योतिष, गणित, धर्म, राजनीति, हस्तिविद्या, अश्वविद्या, आयुर्वेद, धनुर्वेद, गान्धर्ववेद, योग, वाणिज्य, चित्रकला, शिल्पकला, वास्तुकला, नृत्य, नाट्य, काव्य and several other *Vidyās* and *Kalās*. These works continue to stand as the memorable and concrete embodiments of the manifold expressions of their inquisitive intellect, ably assisted by their irresistible enthusiasm. Their analytical intellect was never averse to any subject under the sky. There is no subject under the sun on which something has not been written in Sanskrit. The people in general, and the intellectuals in particular, were so very scientific minded that they could not think of virtuosity as a bar to the scientific investigation of any subject.

Someśvara III was not only a king, but a royal adviser, a religious teacher, a great educationist, a great philosopher and a great well-wisher of mankind. As such, his work Rāja Mānasollāsa is useful and interesting not only to the common people but also to those who want more than the worldly things. It may be said that it is one of the most important works in Sanskrit literature.

Rāja Mānasollāsa written in Anuṣṭubh metre, is interspersed with prose passages. Its language is easy but florid. The work treats of many subjects and gives maximum information. The work is designated by the author as the "जगदाचार्यपुस्तकः" or a book which teaches the world. The scope of the book is so extensive that it can rightly claim that epithet.

Rāja Mānasollāsa is a well-known encyclopaedic work in Sanskrit literature composed in verses by Someśvara III (1127-38 A.D.), a distinguished scholar. He was the son of the great king Vikramāditya VI. Someśvara proved to be a monumental figure in the history of Cālukyas, who ruled at Kalyāṇa in Karnāṭaka (India), from the 10th to the end of the 12th century. Rāja Mānasollāsa contains elaborate information on almost all branches of ancient lores. Hence, it serves as a storehouse of information on all leading topics of learning. This interesting work is useful to the common man to lead a peaceful life. Rāja Mānasollāsa propounds time-tested knowledge, and accordingly, gives fresh inspiration to human beings even in the present day changing times. It consists of five *Prakaraṇās* of twenty chapters each of unequal length and encompasses several related subjects.

General topics are explained in the first *Prakaraṇa.* They are : general and religious ethics, social service, manufacture of idols, diseases and their remedies. In the second *Prakaraṇa,* polity is treated in detail under seven different heads. Law, both personal and interstate, and other aspects such as peace, war, invasion, neutrality and alliance, are also dealt with. The third *Prakaraṇa* is devoted to the description with minutest details, of architecture, picture-drawing, painting, iconography and the pleasure of domestic life. The fourth and fifth *Prakaraṇas* explain the various forms of amusements and entertainments. Incidentally, a brief reference is also made to arithmetic, decimal notations, preparation of calendars, astrology, omens, augury, palmistry, training of horses and elephants along with the treatment of their diseases, mining, alchemy, gems and precious stones, marriage and child-rearing, cookery, liquor, beverages, music, conveyances, scents, and so on.

The subjects treated in Rāja Mānasollāsa give a bird's eye view of social services, ethics, education, health, justice and the role of a physician in the welfare state. Education, imparted with devotion and dedication, enables a society to be mentally alert to face the increasing challenges posed by the changing times. Health, meticulously guarded, keeps the society physically fit and mentally calm and peaceful to utilise all energies for the well-being of mankind. The place of a physician in the establishment is highlighted by Someśvara in a befitting manner. He opines that the well-being of a State depends upon mental, physical and social health of its subjects. Mental health depends upon the imparting of all-round education aimed at intellectual, emotional and spiritual advancement of all people. Physical health is assured by taking timely precautions in warding off diseases. Social health is assured by the dispensation of speedy and impartial justice without fear or favour.

The ruler of a kingdom, according to Rāja Mānasollāsa, should regard the protection of health, wealth and progress of his people on a priority basis. There should be adequate facilities for guarding the people against all sorts of pollution so that their mental, physical and moral health is assured. There should be enough opportunities for the people to make an honest living through hard work. Health is also wealth in a strict sense. Only healthy people can utilise their energy for increasing the wealth of a state. They alone can ensure steady economic growth and make the country prosperous. With this object in view, Someśvara gives a place of prominence to physicians in society to enable them to discharge their duties and to rid society of various types of diseases. The king is visualizing an ideal society in which diseases related to human beings as well as animals have to be diagnosed and treated by his physicians and doctors.

Kshemendrā in his 'Auchityavichāracharchā', has stressed the importance of freedom from pollution. He points out that there are five types of pollution : (i) Pollution of the mind; (ii) Pollution of action; (iii) Pollution of family; (iv) Pollution of body; and (v) Pollution of speech. He considers pollution of the mind as the most depressing.

In the present century, we are living in an era of pollution of all types. Prevention of pollution is an uphill task facing mankind. The sages of yore had a vision of life. They strongly pleaded for preventing the mind from being polluted. If the mind is purified, they argued, other types of environmental pollution can be minimised, if not totally eliminated. This is possible by mind-control. Mind-control depends upon cultivation of pure habits in thought, word and deed.

Someśvara's family boasts of eminent scholars who had made significant contribution to the cause of Sanskrit learning and had been befittingly honoured for their scholarship, right from his forefather Taila (Tailapa) II, who ruled around 973 A.D. After the extinction of the Bādāmi Cālukyas in Karnāṭaka in 757 A.D., there was a gap of two centuries, after which a branch of the Eastern Cālukya dynasty came to power in the tenth century, only to fall again in 1198 A.D. With the death of the last chief of the line of Someśvara IV, Tailapa II, founded the Cālukya dynasty in Karnāṭaka. This dynasty was just an offshoot of the Bādāmi Cālukyas. He established his Kingdom with Halasige (in Belgaum District) as his capital.[1] Tailapa II, was a subordinate of Kṛṣṇa III. In 957 A.D. we find him as a subordinate of Kannaradeva, governing the Melapati region. But later, in a record of 965 A.D., he is mentioned as a *Mahāsāmanta,* governing *Tardavadi* 1,000 division. In this record, he is given the titles 'Cālukyarāma' and 'Āhavamalla' and described as 'Satyāśraya-kula-tilaka'.[2] This indicates the rise of his power and influence. He ruled for 24 years from 973 to 997 A.D. He was an able warrior and overcame with determined effort the many obstacles that came to him on his way to secure and stabilise his new kingdom. He declared himself as the 'Lion of Cālukyās'.[3] Thereafter, the dynasty continued for some years later.

This dynasty was fortunate to have five great warriors and statesmen, rulers of eminence in unbroken succession, viz., Taila II, Satyāśraya, Jayasiṁha, Someśvarā I and Vikramāditya VI. This advantage raised the status, prestige and influence of this dynasty in the southern part of India. Among all these kings, Vikramāditya VI, became very famous. We find that the period of fifty years of rule of Vikramāditya VI, was one of uninterrupted peace. Krishna Murāri[4] says : "Vikramāditya then entered Kalyāṇa and had a long, and on the whole, a peaceful reign of fifty years. It does not, however, mean that there were no disturbances at all. In fact, his younger brother and Yuvarāja Jayasiṁha, was the first to raise a revolt against Vikramāditya's rule. Jayasiṁha no doubt supported him earlier in ousting the elder brother. For this he was suitably rewarded by the new king who appointed him Yuvarāja. During his father's life-time Jayasiṁha was the governor of *Tardavādi* division in 1064 A.D., when Someśvara II came to the throne." All this shows that Jayasiṁha was highly regarded by his elder brother and king who had great confidence in him. Vikramāditya VI was a great soldier, and his early training was directed towards making him a through warrior and good citizen. It is no wonder that he possessed a sturdy physique and outstanding administrative skill. He was not only a great soldier but a wise statesman and a skilled diplomat also. I.M. Muthanna says : "Cālukya Vikrāma VI, was an equally great ruler who went as far as Bengal and Assam and later towards Kerala and Simhala in the south."[5] After a long rule of fifty years, Vikramāditya VI, passed away early in 1127 A.D. He has left behind a number of inscriptions which give us useful information about the various aspects of life of the people in that period. An inscription from Āland affirms that under the beneficial rule of this monarch, the Kali (iron) age was transformed into Kṛta (golden) age.[6]

We learn from Vikramāditya VI's inscriptions that he had about a dozen wives and four sons. Queen Candalādevī was the mother of Someśvara III, Jayakarana and Tailapa. Mallikārjuna who figures as Yuvarāja governing the *Tardavādi* division and the Karahāḍa 4,000 was also probably a son of Candalādevī. She was a princess of the Śilāhāra family of Karahāḍa, who wooed the Cālukya king in a "Svayaṁvara" as described by Bilhaṇa.[7] She is described in a number of records as a lady of exceptional accomplishments. The epithets, "Nṛtya Vidyādharī" i.e., an adept in the art of dancing[8] and Abhinava-Sarasvatī, or Abhinava-Śāradā,[9] ascribed to her appear to be more factual than formal, indicative of her proficiency in music, dance and other fine arts. Among the other queens, mention may be made of Ketaladevī, Malayamatīdevī, Padmalādevī and queen Jakalādevī who was a pious lady and a follower of Jaina faith. Some of them were good administrators. Taila III, viewing with concern the growing menance to his kingdom, had appointed for some time in about 1158 A.D., (1162-1198 A.D.) his son Tribhuvanamalla Someśvara IV as his successor and invested him with sovereign powers. But this prince, with probably two other princes of the family, fled to a safe place to escape from the hands of Bijjala who was succeeding in his aggressive plans.

Someśvara gives in his 'Vikrāmānkabhyudaya', some information about the heredity of his family. According to him, Taila II had three sons by name Satyāśraya,[10] Daśavarman, and Pulakeśī. Then Jayasiṁha II had a son by name Āhavamalla. Further, he mentions that Vikramāditya VI was known to be the greatest ruler in the Cālukya dynasty. As noted above, historians opine that Vikramāditya VI had four sons by name Mallikārujna, Someśvara, Jayakarna, and Tailapa. This information is contained in the inscriptions found near Basavakalyāṇa.

In Kalyāṇa dynasty, Tailapa, Iriva Bedaṅga, Someśvara I and Vikramāditya VI occupied the Telugu areas. They fought with the Colās also. Vijayapura was the capital of the Cālukyas of Kalyāṇa.[11] Lakkundi or Lakkingundi was a great centre at that time and Kalyāṇapuri was famous in many ways. According to Krishna Murāri,[12] "Towards the close of the tenth century the power of the Rāṣṭrakūṭas waned, and the main line of the Cālukyas which emerged from obscurity of about two centuries, once more dominated the political scene of the Deccan with Kalyāṇapuri, 'the best of all the cities in the world' as their capital contesting the sovereignty of India, South of the Vindhyas with the Colas of the Tamil country. War and politics were by no means the only concern of the Cālukyas. They figured prominently as patrons of art and learning. They were great builders, and one dominant style of Indian architecture derives its name from them. Kannada and Telugu literatures drew sustenance from their patronage." Bilhaṇa and the jurist Vijñāneśvara of the Mitākṣara code lived at Kalyāṇa. During the time of the Cālukyas, Karnāṭaka became a great power which contributed to the cultural greatness of India. The restoration of Cālukya supremacy inaugurated a new era of architectural renaissance, wherein came forth a sumptuous harvest of glorious monuments.[13] According to P.B. Desai, "This period may therefore be described as a golden period as vouched by a large number of inscriptions found in these areas."[14]

Vikramāditya VI had left nothing to be achieved afresh by his successors. Added to this, Someśvara III was a person of a different bent of mind. He was more a scholar than a fighter. Generally speaking, the reign of Vikramāditya VI was a period of happiness for the Deccan. He founded a new town named Vikramapura.[15] Vikramāditya VI was succeeded by his son Someśvara III in A.D. 1127. He was as great a monarch as his father. But he was greater than his father in one respect; being a learned man himself, he bore the title 'Bhūlokamalla', 'the wrestler of the earth' and 'Sarvajña Cakravarti', 'the omniscient emperor'. Fortunately for him, there were no notable disturbances inside the country or on the borders. Therefore, valuable books like Rāja Mānasollāsa or Abhilaṣitārtha Ciṁtāmaṇī and *Vikramānkābhyudayam* could be written.

The scholarly and voluminous work Rāja Mānasollāsa running into about 8,000 verses, is divided into five *Viṁśatis* or *Prakaraṇas,* each containing twenty *Adhyāyas* or chapters of unequal length, some chapters again comprising of several sub-sections.

As a philosopher, poet, and as a great political thinker, Someśvara III occupies a pre-eminent position. In this way, he may be said to have excelled his forefathers in the breadth of the spectrum of activities. According to B.R. Gopal[16], "Bhūlokamalla's rule of about 13 years was one of peace in the kingdom." "Someśvara's pious nature and interest in academic pursuits had resulted in peace and harmony in the kingdom. Political sagacity, selfless devotion and respect for his elders and preceptors,[17] unshakable faith in Lord Śiva[18] and Viṣṇu,[19] and remarkable foresight are a few among his numerous virtues.

The *Arthaśāstra* of Kauṭilya is a monumental work on polity, which refers to previous discussions and in some respects attempts a comparative study of the subject. Kauṭilya quotes the following individuals or schools of opinion, viz., Manu, Uśanas, Bṛhaspati, Bharadvāja, Viśālākṣa, Kauṇapadanta, Paraśara and Bahudantiputra, etc. There are other works which are more or less representative of their times and throw much light on the subject by their mass of information. But we should draw not merely upon these treatises, or those portions of them that deal specifically with polity, but also upon others which, though not directly treating it, throw many hints and side-lights, the combined effect of which may clear up many an obscure corner of the subject of our inquiry.

Political realism believes that politics, like society in general, is governed by objective laws that have their roots in human nature. In order to improve society, it is necessary to understand first the laws which govern the society. The operation of these laws being rigid, men will challenge them only at the risk of failure. It is generally believed that human nature has not changed much since the classical period. Hence, novelty is not necessarily a virtue in political theory, nor is old age a defect. The fact that a theory of politics, if there be such a theory, has never been heard of before, tends to create a presumption against, rather than in favour of its soundness. Conversely, the fact that a theory of politics developed hundreds or even thousands of years ago, as was the theory of the balance of power, does not create a presumption that it must be outmoded and obsolete. A theory of politics must be subjected to the dual test of reason and experience. To dismiss such a theory because it had its flowering in centuries past is to present not a rational argument but a modernistic prejudice that takes for granted the superiority of the present over the past.

The maxims relating to polity and statecraft, expounded in chapter II of Rāja Mānasollāsa have been discussed frequently. Most of them conform to the traditional pattern. *Rājadharma, Daṇḍanīti* and the importance of the ministers, Treasury, Fort,

Ally, *Purohita, Yuvarāja, Senāpati, Dvārapāla, Āntarveśika, Kārāgārādhyakṣa, Nagarādhyakṣa, Dharmādhyakṣa, Sabhādhyakṣa, Daṇḍapāla* and *Durgapāla,* etc., occupy the bulk of the space.

The Rāja Mānasollāsa refers to three Śaktis or powers that operate in a state. They are *Utsāhaśakti,* the personal energy and drive of the ruler himself, *Prabhuśakti,* the power of the army and treasury, and *Mantraśakti,* the power of counsel and diplomacy.[20] These powers are thought of in connection with a state's relations with other states and have no bearing on the internal structure of a state's organisation.

King's Power and Functions

The power and functions of the king as laid down in the *Smṛtis, Arthaśāstra* and *Kāmandakīya Nītisāra,* do not in any way differ from what we find in the Rāja Mānasollāsa. During the reign of king Someśvara, there were rulers in other regions, who were not autocrats. They were fully conscious of their responsibilities and duties to the state and their subjects. The realization of *Trivarga* was an ideal of a state. The king was advised to follow *Dharma, Artha* and *Kāma* in their moderate limitations without injuring the interests of one another. The first duty of the king was to protect his subjects as his own children.[21] Someśvara has mentioned in great detail the religious duties of a king without deviating from the hereditary point of view. Someśvara had constructed many works of public utility. He was a great builder in every sense of the term, builder of a great empire and a brave army. His rule, therefore, resulted in prosperity, peace and plenty. Buildings, which have architectural value, will be referred to later. Here, we may note that he constructed reservoirs, tanks and irrigation canals for the welfare of his subjects. By protecting the *Svadharma* of his subjects, the king fulfilled *Trivarga. Svadharma* is the particular duty of each individual in every group. Though Someśvara on the whole acknowledges *Svadharma,* yet he mentions *Samāna-Dharma,* the duties common to all castes and groups. Someśvara discusses them in the Rāja Mānasollāsa in the first *Prakaraṇa.* These are kindness, truthfulness, not aspiring for other's property, controlling one's desires, avoiding marriage against the order of the castes and chastity. The king's duty is to promote these practices among his subjects. By protecting *Svadharma* of his subjects, the king receives one sixth of the fruit of the religious merit of his subjects.

Importance of Flora in Rāja Mānasollāsa

Someśvara exhibits his vast knowledge of horticulture. A description of various methods employed for the care and maintenance of trees and plants bears testimony to this fact. He refers to trees bearing fruits. He describes various types of trees as follows :

1. *Citraphala Vṛkṣāḥ* i.e., trees bearing strange fruits.
2. *Phalabhūyiṣṭhāḥ* i.e., trees bearing abundant fruits.
3. *Sarvakālaphalānvitāḥ* i.e., trees which bear fruits throughout the year.
4. *Svāduphalopetāḥ* i.e., trees bearing delicious fruits.
5. *Tatkālikaphalodayaḥ* i.e., trees which bear fruits instantly.[22]

Cālukya king Someśvara knows the importance of the trees, and their effects. So he says that much care should be taken of the trees and plants as if they are our own children. (*Putravatpari-pālitaḥ*). Further, he instructs the officers that they must not only increase well-fertilized lands but also take care to maintain good forests. He recommends that the trees—Aśoka, Niṁba, Punnāga, Bakula, Nāgakesara, Śirīṣa and Tilaka—should be planted first in the forest as they bring about happiness, glory and prosperity.[23]

Someśvara tells about watering of trees and plants as

follows : The watering process should differ according to the change of seasons. Then only we get good results in getting desired fruits and flowers. The first thing to be observed in this connection is that for full one year after sowing the seeds, one should water the plants with a *Kumbha* (earthen pot) and the number of the *Kumbhas* should be increased according to the number of years. Someśvara suggests that it should be continued for twenty years.[24] In the *Hemanta* and *Śiśira* seasons, the trees should be watered on alternate days. In *Vasanta* and *Grīṣma,* they should always be watered in the morning. In the *Varṣā* and *Śarad* seasons they should be watered only when the base of the trees is dry.[25]

Someśvara mentions about the treatment of the seeds. Two methods are given in this connection. The first method is applicable to the seeds of all kinds of trees. According to this method, the seeds of ripe fruits are first dried in the sun. Then they are kept covered with cowdung for five days. They are fumigated with the smoke of *Viḍaṅga ghṛta.*[26] The second method is about a special treatment given to the milky trees. According to this method, the seeds are soaked in cow's milk continuously for ten nights. They are dried in shade, coated with cowdung and mixed with the milk of a tigress and ashes and with barley and wheat.[27]

Then he mentions about the treatment of the soil. The soil used for planting fruit and flower giving trees should be sprinkled with sweet water and should be free from pieces of stones. It should be smooth and soft. Someśvara says that the following should be used as manure for getting the highest yield : (1) Dung of pigs, horses, etc. (2) Fats of elephant, fox, deer, etc. (3) Flesh of fish, dog, mouse, deer, cat, cāṣa bird etc.[28] (5.1.40-98). Further, he tells about pits. The pit in which a tree is to be planted should be four feet square and four feet deep. The trees should be planted according to their size. They may be of big, medium or small size. The space between the trees should accordingly be about 16, 11, 8 or 14 *hastas*[29] (one *hasta* measures about 18 inches).

Trees and plants should be well protected from frost, extreme heat, smoke, fire, insects and birds. Weeds should not be allowed to grow near the pits.[30] He further suggests some other methods to protect the trees. Trees should be protected against snowfall.[31] The insects and worms can also be killed if *Viḍaṅga, Hiṅgu Sindhūra, Marica, Ativiṣa, Vacā, Bhallātaka* and the (powdered) horn of a buffalow are mixed in equal quantities into the soil. This process cures all the diseases of the plants.[32] In this way, king Someśvara discusses about the science dealing with plant life. The third chapter of this thesis discusses about the science dealing with the life of humans as also of animals. Thus, it can be seen that Someśvara is well-versed in the science of living organisms.

Geographic Study in Rāja Mānasollāsa

The knowledge of Geography of Someśvara reveals a general resemblance with that of Kālidāsa, Bāṇa and Bhāravi with reference to the concept of different geographical units and divisions of Ancient Bhārata. These writers were separated by more than 1,000 years and belonged to different parts of the land. These writers show acquaintance with the regions to which they did not belong, though it must be admitted that their description of the regions of their nativity is more precise and hence authentic. But some writers derive a considerable number of topographical details from the common source, the Purāṇas, which Someśvara consults or refers more frequently and profusely in case of rivers and mountains, etc. This fact partly explains the similarity of geographical data found in works of some writers. This is due also to the fact that the geographical names were rarely disturbed in ancient times, even though changes took place quite often in the political field. These changes, however, did affect the boundaries of different states and *Janapadas*. It is worthwhile to note that a good number of old geographical names are still current either in identical form or in a slightly changed form, and this fact facilitates the otherwise difficult task of identifying the ancient places.

Someśvara as a Poet

Someśvara is hailed as the Prince among Indian Poets. Individuals may equal or excel him in one or other aspects of the art of composing poems. But collectively taken, in all aspects, he is unequalled. His uniformly high excellence of style is all his own, not to be found elsewhere in his time. The perfect balance of sound and sense is incomparable. The ease with which he uses words that literally flow from his brilliant mind (*Pratibhā Śakti*) is bewildering. He is a close observer of all kinds of men and their nature. His insight into the human mind is deep and characterisation life-like. As a poet of human nature, he is very famous for his dazzling descriptions, sharing the joys and griefs, feelings and emotions of humanity, charming *Svabhāvoktis,* etc. He has a keen sense of humour and a very healthy optimistic outlook and zeal for life. From the analysis of the contents of the Rāja Mānasollāsa, it is seen that Someśvara deals with all factors connected with human life. Lastly, Someśvara suggests to the kings that they must give sufficient wealth to the good poets and logicians.[33] Because of such benevolence and encouragement, literature of eternal value came to be produced in abundance during those days.

Someśvara knew the importance of the words and their meaning very well. Hence he was able to bring out a better elaboration of different figures of speech easily. Also notable in his *Kāvya* are the different styles and the striking expressions.

As a literary artist, Someśvara stands second to none. His language is natural, simple, chaste and refined. His thoughts and ideas are so profound that they make one infer that he must have had liberal education in a systematic manner. His imaginative faculty is wonderful and sentiments lofty. His work Rāja Mānasollāsa suggests clearly that in his early life he must have spared no pains to widen his intellectual capacity and to develop his all-round knowledge. It has been already shown how it is evident from the study of his work that he had mastered thoroughly all the scriptures and the works in different branches of Sanskrit learning.

Someśvara had mastery over the works of great scholars like Viśvakarma, Maya and Piṅgalācārya. He had studied the *Matsya Purāṇa* also.[34] He had studied the Vedas with their auxiliary works as well as the *Śāstras*. His works bear ample testimony to the same. He was well-grounded in the Rāmāyaṇa, the Mahābhārata, as well as in the *Purāṇas*.[35]

In this way, Someśvara has included several branches of knowledge in Rāja Mānasollāsa. So, this work is rightly considered to be an encyclopaedia. He himself says that he was *Garbhasārasvateya,* i.e., scholar from birth. This statement is not an exaggeration at all. Further, he advises the kings that they must keep their *Prajā* or people always happy, for which the kings must study the work Rāja Mānasollāsa. Rāja Mānasollāsa is written for the sake of *Prajārañjana*. Here he gives the example of the moon. According to Someśvara, just as the moon gives pleasure to mankind by moonlight, Rāja Mānasollāsa does so by the rich knowledge embodied in it. Hence, he has very rightly said that the kings must study Rāja Mānasollāsa in the interest of the welfare of their subjects. He also suggests that scholars also should study this work for the development of their knowledge.[36] The author's skill in collecting, editing, composing and presenting the matter is superb. Hence, Rāja Mānasollāsa caters to the needs of people of all classes. This proves that Someśvara's contribution to knowledge is undoubtedly unique and invaluable. Noting all these things, the reader of Rāja Mānasollāsa will feel to have gained something of everything.

References

1. I.M. Muthanna, *Karnataka History, Administration and Culture* (Bangalore, 1977), p. 61.
2. P.B. Desai (Ed.), *A History of Karnataka*. Dharwad, K.R.I., 1981). p. 159.
3. Krishna Murāri, *The Cālukyas of Kalyani,* Concept Publishing Company, Delhi 1977, p. 41.
4. *Ibid.*, p. 122.
5. I.M. Muthanna, *op.cit.* p. 53.
6. P.B. Desai (Ed.), *op.cit.* p. 185.
7. *Ibid.*
8. V.S. Kulkarni, "Historical and Cultural Studies of the Region Around Basavakalyan" Ph.D. Thesis, Karnatak University, Dharwad, 1979, p. 53.
9. P.B. Desai, *op.cit.* p. 185.
10. The Name of Satyāśraykula is derived from that of one of the early Cālukya kings—Satyaśrī, or Satyāśraya. (cf. *Indian Antiquary*, Jas Burgess, Vol. I. 1872, p. 141).
11. Krishna Murāri. *The Cālukyas of Kalyāṇi*, Concept Publishing Comapny, Delhi, 1977, p. 151.
    cf. A.S. Nanjundaswami. *History of Cālukya*. (in Kannada) (Samaja Book Depot, Dharwad, 1976), p. 47. Cf. I.M. Muthanna. *op.cit.* p. 62.
12. Krishna Murāri, *op.cit.* p. 1.
13. P.B. Desai. *op.cit.* p. 212.
14. *Ibid.*, p. 193.
15. Krishna Murāri. *op.cit.* p. 147.
16. B.R. Gopal, *The Cālukyas of Kalyana and the Kalachuris*, Prasaranga, Karnatak University, Dharwad, 1981, p. 314.
17. असूयावर्जनं चैव पतितैः संगवर्जनम्।
    क्रोधस्य वर्जनं चैव स्वात्मस्तुतिविवर्जनम्।। (1.1.15)
    पितृणां तर्पणं कार्यमतियेश्चैव भोजनम्।
    शुश्रूषणं गुरूणां च तपस्तीर्थेषु मज्जनम्।। (1.1.17)
18. वन्दे भवलताबीजं लिंगरूपं महेश्वरम्।
    अव्यक्तमपि सुव्यकं यस्यान्तः सचराचरम्।। (1.1.3)
19. नौमि वेदध्वनिवरं देवं धत्ते सदैव हि।
    नाभिपद्मोदरे विष्णोः क्रणद्भ्रमरविभ्रमम्।। (1.1.5)
    सुदर्शनदलितबाणबाहो शिरोमात्रावशेषीकृतराहो
    निरवधिशास्त्रार्थोपदेशदक्ष संगररंगदलितहिरण्याक्ष।
    समुत्सारितपुरन्दर भयविहित-प्रणतजनपापक्षय
    संसारपारावार-सन्तरणसेतो जय जय नाथ वैनतेयकेतो।। (4.16.357)

20. षड् गुणा: शक्तयस्तिस्र: प्रभावोत्साहमन्त्रजा:।
भेदो दण्ड: साम दानमित्युपायचतुष्टयम्।। (अमरकोश:, 1.1.22)
21. स्वराष्ट्रे पालयेद्राजा प्रजा: पुत्रानिवौरसान्।
चोरेभ्योऽमात्यकेभ्यश्य तथैवार्थाधिकारित:।। (2.3.155.)
22. तत्र चित्रद्रुमोपेतं वनं कुर्यात्समन्तत:। तन्मध्ये रुचिरं रम्यं क्रीडाहेतोर्मनोहरम्।।
कारयेत्पर्वतं राजा तुङ्गशृङ्गविराजितम्। नानावृक्ष-समाकीर्णं सुविशालशिलातलम्।।
तत्र चित्रफला वृक्षात्तत्प्रयोगविनिर्मिता:। अन्यपत्रान्यफलका: पुत्रवत्परिपालिता:।।
अनन्तफलभूयिष्ठा: सर्वकाल फलान्विता:। लाघवोऽपि महाकाया: प्रशस्ता: कुब्जातं गता:।।
अन्ये स्वादुफलोपेतास्तात्कालिकफलोदया:। प्रयत्नेने कृता: शैले नाना फलमहीरुहा:।।
(5.1.2.6.)
23. अशोकनिम्बपुन्नागबकुला नागकेसर:।
शिरीषस्तिलकश्चैवमुप्यन्ते प्रथमं वने।।
सुखारोग्य यशोवृद्धिलक्ष्मीविजय वृद्धये।
सौभाग्यार्थमिमे वृक्षा: कर्तव्या भूभृता वने।। (5.1.18-19)
24. बीजावापात्समारभ्य कुम्भेनेकेन सेचयेत्।
यावद्वर्षं तत: कुम्भं प्रतिवर्षं विवर्धयेत्।।
समानां विंशतिर्यावत्ततस्तेनैव मानत:।
जलं देयं प्रयत्नेन यथाकालं महीरूहान्।। (5.1.33-34)
25. हेमन्ते शिशिरे देयं तोयमेकान्तरे दिने।
वसन्ते च तथा ग्रीष्मे देयं प्रात: सदा बुधै:।।
वर्षासु च शरत्काले यदा शुष्कं महीतलम्।
तदा देयं जलं तज्ज्ञैरालवाले महीरुहाम्।। (5.1.21-22)
26. स्वभावपक्वफलिनोर्निर्दोषं शुष्कमातपे।
फलबीजं समालिप्तं गोमये दिनपञ्चकम्।।
विडङ्गघृतधूपेन धूपितं कारयेद्भृशम्।
सर्वेषामेव वृक्षाणामेष बीजविधि: स्मृत:।। (5.1.7-8)
27. गोक्षीरभावितं बीजं दशरात्रं निरन्तरम्।
छायाशुष्कं च मिलितं व्याघ्रीदुग्धेन भस्मना।।
यवगोधूममिलितं गोमयेन प्रलेपितम्।
स्थापयेत् क्षीरवृक्षाणां विधेया बीजसंस्कृति:।। (5.1.9-10)
28. द्राक्षा भवति सुस्वादुर्भूयिष्ठ-फलशोभिता। (5.1.42)
29. षोडशैकादशाष्टौ वा तथा हस्ताश्चतुर्दश।
कर्तव्यं रोप्यमाणानामन्तरालं महीरहाम्।। (5.1.13)
30. नीहाराच्चण्डतापाच्च धूमाद्वैश्वानरात्तथा।
जालकारा: (रात्) प्रयत्नेन रक्षणीया: क्षमारुह:। (5.1.25)
31. विद्युता दग्धवृक्षस्य भूमिमादायनन्दने।
रक्षार्थिं विक (कि) रेद्रेषां तया न हिमबाधनम्।। 5.1.27)

32. विहङ्गहिङ्गुसिन्धूत्थमरिचातिविषावचाः।
भल्लातकं तथा शृङ्गं माहिषं समभागतः।।
एतैर्विरचितो योगै निहन्यात् क्रि (कृ) मिकीटकम्।
उद्याने पादपानां तु सर्वव्याधिविनाशनः।। (5.1.31-32)

33. कवीनां तार्किकाणाञ्च प्रसादं भूरि दापयेत्।
उक्तः शास्त्रविनोदोऽयं सोमेश्वरमहीभुजा।। (4.2.404)

34. विश्वकर्म-मतेनापि मयशास्त्रानुसारतः।
मत्स्यप्रोक्तविधानेन पिङ्गलामतमानतः।। (1.11.76)

35. शृङ्गारोदधिशीतांशून् रागाम्बुजदिवाकरान्।
कथां पृच्छेन्महीपालो महाभारत-सम्भवाम्।।
रामायणोद्भवां भव्यां पुराणेभ्यः समुद्गताम्।
बृहत्कथा समुत्पन्नां वीराणां चरितोत्कटाम्।। (4.19.1411-1412)

36. राज्यप्राप्तेर्नृपकुलभुवामित्युपायोपदेशः
सम्यक् सोमेश्वरनृपतिना गर्भसारस्वतेन।
चक्रे चन्द्रप्रातिमयशसा रञ्जनाय प्रजानां
पुण्यौधानामपि च महतां वृद्धये बुद्धये च।। (1.20.308)

2

ANCIENT TREATISES ON ĀYURVEDA

An effort has been made in this chapter to understand the concepts of ancient Indian medicine system (Āyurveda). Someśvara has, in the Rāja Mānasollāsa, stated "वैद्यशास्त्रानुसारेण कारयेत् तत्प्रतिक्रियाम्।।" (1.19.143). In the light of this statement, it becomes clear that Someśvara had acquired full knowledge of ancient Indian medicine system or Āyurveda or life science system.

King Someśvara has presented the concepts on how to lead a peaceful life, mentioned in the Sanskrit texts, which were written centuries ago. Many of these concepts are valid even today. Every person desires to achieve knowledge, brilliance of mind, wealth, strength and robust health. For this purpose King Someśvara prays as follows :

शौर्यं धैर्यं क्षमौदार्यं शुचित्वं प्रियवादिता।
उद्योगित्वमनिर्वेदः सर्वदा धर्मकारिता।।
जनानुरागः सौभाग्यं शास्त्रशस्त्रास्त्र नैपुणम्।
विवेको दृढचित्तत्वं कलाकुशलता धनम्।। 2.1.4-5

Here, the performance of proper duty is suggested. It is known that a person blessed with a healthy mind in healthy body is able to lead a successful life. Our age-old prayer to God has been that we should not be tempted to indulge in deceitful activities and God should lead us to render useful service to the community. Caraka also expresses precisely the same thoughts as follows : बुद्धि सिद्धिः स्मृतिर्मेधा धृति कीर्तिः क्षमा दया।। (चरकसंहिता- सूत्रस्थान-1.39). Ṛgveda declares (8-12-19) that "Gods are propitiated and their vigour enhanced by prayer and praise".

Medical treatises of Caraka and Suśruta, which represent the earliest extant books on Āyurveda, clearly indicate that this form of medicine has never completely disappeared, but was probably superseded over time by a system of medicine based on empirical-rational principles and practices, issuing from an active encounter with the world. It should not be assumed that empiricism or the process of observing and defining is evident only in the classical medical tradition. Vedic medicine relied on close observation of phenomena in order to develop its unique form of mythical and religious classifications and associations. The difference between these two epistemologies lies in their respective premises. The foundation of Vedic medicine was a belief in a multitude of benevolent and malevolent deities or spirits that populated the cosmos and caused good and bad effects in the human realm. Controlling and taming these entities were the ultimate goals of this healing system. In Āyurveda, a basic understanding of the interrelation-ship between human-beings and their environment prefaced every observation. Ideally, human-beings and nature should be in perfect harmony. Disease occurred when the equilibrium between these two was disrupted. Restoration of a fundamental balance was the goal of this medical system.

The social event occurring in Vedic antiquity was probably a key factor in initiating change. A forthright denigration of medicine by the priestly order and the Brahmanic hierarchy resulted in the exclusion of healers from the orthodox ritual cults because of the defilement they incurred from contact with impure people with whom they found fellowship. This type of "excommunication" transformed the medical priests into members of a fringe-group. Other important marginalized people included the heterodox wandering ascetics who renounced the trappings of orthodox ideologies and practices and abandoned society for the wilderness in search of higher spiritual goals. Unencumbered by the strictures of Brahmanical orthodoxy, these ascetics, who included among others the Buddhists, acquired a radically different view of the world and mankind's place in it, fostered by their intense meditative discipline. In fact, early Buddhist literature reveals that their understanding of the relationship between human beings and nature was not very different from that which contributed to Āyurvedic medical thought. An intellectual sympathy seemingly was shared by both the wandering ascetics on a spiritual quest and the roving physicians whose professional curiosity led them to encounters with different sorts of people from whom they could obtain useful medical knowledge.

Finding rapport with the communities of heterodox ascetics and renunciants who were not inclined to censure their philosophies, practices and associations, the healers, like the knowledge-seeking ascetics, wandered the countryside performing cures and acquiring ever new remedies, treatment and medical information. They eventually became practically indistinguishable from the mendicants with whom they were in close contact. A vast storehouse of medical knowledge soon developed among these wandering physicians who, like the ascetics, were unhindered by Brahmanic strictures and taboos. With the help of ideas from the intellectual ascetics, the physicians began to conceive a radically new epistemology with which to codify and systematize this body of efficacious medical data.

Fitting into the Buddha's key teaching of the middle way between worldly indulgence and self-denial, medicine became part of Buddhism by providing the means to maintain a healthy bodily state characterized by an equilibrium—both within the body and between the body and its surroundings. Portions of the repository of medical lore were codified in the early monastic rules, thereby giving rise to a Buddhist monastic medical tradition. The early Buddhist community of monks or *saṅgha* was where wandering intellectuals would gather and exchange information which often included medical knowledge. As the *saṅgha* established more permanent dwellings and fixed abodes for ascetics, the intellectual life turned more scholarly, and a formal systematization of information and instruction ensued. The symbiotic relationship between Buddhism and medicine in the large conglomerate monasteries (*vihāras*) expedited the acceptance of Buddhism in other parts of Asia. Probably during the early centuries of the common era, Brāhmaṇism assimilated the storehouse of medical knowledge into its socio-religious traditions.

The most fascinating study in Āyurveda is its history from the earliest times in India.

The earliest teacher of Āyurveda is Bhāradwaja and his period is mentioned as Pre-Vedic or Vedic. He is mentioned as having performed severe penance over a long period at the end of which Bhāradwaja went to Indra. At the time of creation, Brahma (creator) is reported to have handed down Āyurveda to Prajāpati who in turn taught it to Aśvinikumārs. Indra is supposed to have received the same from Aśvinikumārs.

After *Kṛtayuga*, the sages purified by penance are said to have assembled in the Himalayas. There is a long list of *Ṛṣis* assembled there to discuss about the welfare of human beings. The most prominent among them were Angiras, Jamadagni, Vaśiṣṭa, Kaśyapa, Bhṛgu, Atreya, Bhāradwaja, Vāmadeva and Mārkaṇḍeya. Prakṛti-equilibrium was considered the basis of *Dharma, Artha, Kāma* and *Mokṣa. Vikṛti,* disequilibrium, was regarded as disorder or disease. Eradication of diseases formed the pivotal point of discussion. They all meditated on Lord Indra who enlightened them about the remedies for the diseases.

The sages decided to send Bhāradwaja as their representative to Indra to know more about the cure for diseases. Indra is reported to have revealed in brief the essence of Āyurveda to him. Bhāradwaja learnt from him the three sutras—हेतु—Reason for diseases, लिंग—Characteristics of diseases and ज्ञान treatment of diseases.[1]

The knowledge received from Indra enabled Bhāradwaja to enjoy longevity in life. He communicated to the rest of the sages this science of life—आयुर्वेद. They came to know the significance of action and reaction of medicines in general as well as special treatment of diseases. The sages enlightened Punarvasu about this extraordinary science of life. He in course of time taught his students, prominent among whom were Agniveśa, Bhela, Jāthukarma, Parāśara, Hārītha and Kśārapāṇi.

The *Tantra-Saṁhitā* was the earliest work brought out by Agniveśa. Bhela followed him by bringing out his *Bhela-Tantra.* Bhela conveyed the same to Punarvasu. The sages were all happy over the achievement of Agniveśa and Bhela. They congratulated them in general and Agniveśa in particular.

Caraka incorporated the salient features of Agniveśa's *Tantra-Saṁhitā* in his *Caraka Saṁhitā* which is regarded even today as the perennial source of Āyurvedic medicine. This is supposed to have eight divisions entitled *Śloka, Nidāna, Vimana, Śarīra, Indriya, Chikitsā, Kalpa* and *Siddhi.* Only seventeen chapters of *Cikitsā Sthāna* are available. Caraka could not complete the entire work. Dradhabala, son of Kāpilabhali, is credited to have completed this famous work.

Atreya, a disciple of Bhāradwaja, is reported to be another reputed teacher of Āyurveda in 8th century B.C.

Patañjali, the author of *Mahābhāṣya,* is credited with having propounded Yoga in the 2nd century B.C. which can effectively remove the dirt of the mind.

It may not be out of context if the anecdote about Caraka is recollected here. It seems Ādiśeṣa came to the earth and saw people were suffering from all types of diseases and were becoming victims of diseases for want of proper treatment. He took pity on such unfortunate human beings. He therefore decided to be born as the son of a sage. He studied the Vedās and Vedāṅgās. No one knew about his presence on the earth where he came as a spy and freely moved about. He became famous as Carakāchārya on the earth and as Vedāchārya in the heavens.[2]

Ādiśeṣa is also credited with having given a separate status to Āyurveda although it formed a part of Atharva Veda.[3]

Suśruta, the earliest surgeon in Āyurveda system, is the renowned author of *Suśruta Saṁhitā* in the 1st century B.C.

An interesting episode about the origin of *Suśruta Saṁhitā* may not be out of place here. It seems king Devodāsa (Dhanvantari in previous birth) was staying at Kāśī in the Vānaprastha stage. Sages approached him and prayed, as follows :

'Oh! my lord! This body is afflicted with *Vāta, Pitta* and *Kapha,* the three evils. *Rajas* and *tamas* also cause mental suffering. Āyurveda is an effective cure for both physical and mental disorder.'

'We pray that you throw light on this aspect for the benefit of mankind, both here and hereafter.'

God Dhanvantari addressed them in this manner : 'Let all of you study Āyurveda. It is called *Aṣṭāṅga.* Please let me know which *Aṅga* should be explained to you.'

The sages replied—'We want to learn Āyurveda with emphasis on *Śalya'*.

The king Devodāsa then explained the first division of *Śalya Tantra* with reference to the four *Pramāṇas—Pratyakṣa, Āgama, Anumāna* and *Upamāna.*[4]

Āyurveda is having eight divisions such as *Kāya, Bala, Graha, Urdhwaṅga, Śalya, Damshtra, Tāra* and *Vrusha.* It is very difficult to study each *Tantra* or Division separately. In order to make it easy for purposes of study, these *Tantras* have been incorporated in eight folds or '*Aṣṭāṅga Saṅgraha*'.[5] *Aṣṭāṅga Hṛdaya* is another masterly work of the age and Vāgbhaṭa is the author who lived in 6th century A.D. He is also mentioned as the compiler of *Aṣṭāṅga Saṅgraha.*

It has been repeatedly mentioned in Āyurveda that the treatment referred to by this 'science of life' is for the benefit of mankind both here and hereafter. Therefore, it is natural to mention Brahman or creator as the first person who knew *Aṣṭāṅga Hṛdaya.* The creator is reported to have taught the same to Prajāpati. It was then made known to Aśvinikumārs and Indra from whom the sage Atri learnt it. Atri handed it over to Agniveśa.[6]

Aṣṭāṅga Hṛdaya Tantras are not in a narrative style. They are in the form of discussion between the sages and the disciples. Agniveśa, the disciple, raises some doubts out of curiosity and the sage Atreya removes his doubts by relevant replies. During the discussion it is made known that reasons for diseases are four-fold, i.e., wind, water, place and time—वायु, जल, देश and काल. Cycle of time or seasonal variation and the rural or urban set up may render both medicine and food lose their taste and effect. Diseases spread on this count. In order to eradicate diseases, food and medicinal plants have to be preserved after thorough scrutiny and proper test.

We must look at Indian medicine rather in terms of distinct phases. Although not well-defined, the first may be called pre-historic or pre-Vedic medicine, dating from about 2700 B.C. to 1500 B.C. The second is that of Vedic medicine which looks back to a time around the second millennium B.C. It is the earliest period in which a clearly discernible medical lore can be ascertained. Vedic medicine is the focus of the present thesis. The next distinguishable stage is characterized by the presence of separate Sanskrit treatises on Indian medical science or Āyurveda, 'the science of longevity.' The earliest of these medical books are the *saṁhitās* of Bhela, Caraka and Suśruta, which date from about the beginning of the Christian era. The subject matter of these works is quite unlike that of Vedic medicine. Most diseases are defined in terms of a humoral theory. According to Indian physicians there are three 'humors' (*doṣas*) : wind (*vāyu),* bile *(pitta)* and phlegm *(kapha, śleṣma*), which on analogy with the humors of the Hippocratic and Galenic systems, were the vitiating forces in the body. (Hippocrates and Galen were great physicians). In a normal state, the humors are in a state of equilibrium in body. When something called a *nidāna,* 'primary cause', which could be of climatic, organic, or less commonly, demonic origin, acted upon the humors, an imbalance occurred, bringing about the manifestation of disease. The principal aim of the physician was to recognize which humor or humors were out of balance and to re-establish the equilibrium through treatments, which usually included drugs with opposite qualities, diet, and daily regimen, although surgery was also sometimes recommended.

This thumbnail sketch of early Āyurvedic medicine serves to illustrate that at its basis lies a theoretical and a rational understanding of disease and cure. The origin of this new approach to medicine is a point of controversy. It is quite certain that a little of it can be traced to Vedic medicine. Although the theoretical framework of Āyurveda may not be Vedic, the basis of its materia medica could indeed have evolved from Vedic medicine or even from pre-historic, pre-Vedic medicine.

A clear and detailed picture of medicine prior to the Vedic phase is difficult to ascertain. Evidence of this pre-historic period in South Asia derives primarily from archaeological remains excavated from the sites of the Harappan culture, sometimes referred to as the Indus Valley Civilization. Its dates are from about 2700 B.C., to 1500 B.C., making it roughly contemporaneous with the old, middle, and new Kingdoms of Egypt and the period of Sumer and Akkad in Mesopotamia. The mosaic of Harappan settlements illustrates a highly developed, urbanized culture, established principally along the Indus river (in Sind, now in Pakistan), stretching from the Arabian sea to as far north as the Panjab (sites have also been found further south in the present-day-Gujarat). The area covered was nearly twice as large as the Egyptian civilization and alomst four times as great as that of Sumer and Akkad.[7] This vast civilization had two main centers or capitals : one in the south, Mohenjodaro (near modern Sukkur) and one in the north, Harappa (near Lahore).

The architecture of the Harappan sites was unique for its time. Streets were planned on a north-south and east-west grid. Houses were usually two-storeyed and made of burnt brick. Many homes contained a bathroom, built near the wall facing the street so that water could be drained through a pipe into a covered sewer running under the street. The bathrooms were either square or rectangular, with a sloping floor with an opening in the corner through which the water could drain. Several of the houses even had latrines with a drainage system similar to that of the bathrooms.[8] These architectural designs point to a conscious concern for public health and sanitation and suggest an implicit belief in ritual purity and pollution, which becomes so prevalent in later Indian thought. The great bath found in the citadel area of Mohenjodaro perhaps epitomizes the Harappan penchant for purification through bathing. The man-made pool measured 108 feet by 180 feet with a centre basin 23 feet by 39 feet and a sloping floor which reached a depth of 8 feet. This giant structure was filled with water from a large well.[9] The central purifying agent was water which, as we shall see, was an important medicine of the Vedic people. It is quite possible, therefore, that hydrotherapy was a therapeutic measure used by the Harappans to restore and to preserve health, which brings to mind the purpose of the Roman baths of a later period.

Unlike the ancient Egyptian and Mesopotamian medical traditions which have specific treatises outlining their medical systems, the earliest Indian textual evidence of medicine is randomly incorporated in the corpora of its principal religious literature, primarily in the Atharvaveda and to a much lesser extent in the Ṛgveda.

The medical material contained in these two ancient texts is not wholly free from problems. Because we have well edited texts with which to work, we stand on fairly firm ground when labouring with these bodies of literature, which have been preserved by an extraordinarily accurate oral tradition from very early times until comparatively recently when they were recorded in written form. Doubts concerning the meaning of specific words and phrases are present; but these uncertainties are not unexpected in such ancient documents. Of all the religious literature of ancient India, these Vedic texts have received the most extensive philological investigation. With this background of scholarship at our disposal, we have a solid basis upon which to test new hypotheses and to construct new theories. Although we may not be able to eliminate all the doubts which the literature still contains, we can, nevertheless, contribute significantly to the elucidation of India's antique medical lore.

The actual medical doctrines we shall study are found mostly in the Atharvaveda, a religious text which contains much material of secular nature. The Ṛgveda is almost entirely religious in character. As such it provides for the most part mythological stories illustrating the healings performed by various gods of the Vedic pantheon.[10] These episodes along with other scattered medical references will be utilized in order to explain more fully the medical philosophy and practice of the Vedic people; but they cannot in themselves be viewed as representing a separate medical tradition. It is only when the two texts are examined together that the fundamental doctrines of the Vedic medical tradition can be fully appreciated.

A work of this type should include a discussion of anatomy. We refrain, however, from an examination of individual anatomical terms, as this has already been undertaken by A.F.R.

Hoernle, F.S. Hammett and especially J. Filliozat, to whose works the reader should refer for the best discussion of the subject.[11] For all their painstaking work on anatomy, Filliozat and the others have neglected to explain adequately the basis of ancient Indian anatomical knowledge.

Anatomical knowledge in ancient India was derived principally from the sacrifice of the horse and of man; chance observations of improperly buried bodies and examinations of the corporal members made by medical men during treatment contributed comparatively little to the body of anatomical knowledge. As a result of the precise ritual procedures of the sacrifice, which called for the recitation of the name of each part of the body as it was cut (for the horse this is documented in Ṛgveda : चतुस्त्रिंशद वाजिनो देवबन्धोर्वङ्कीरश्वस्य स्वधितिः समेति। अच्छिद्रा गात्रा वयुना कृणोत परुष्परुरनुघुष्यावि शस्त्र।। 1.162.18) (for man no early references are found, but later tradition specifies that the action should follow that of the immolation of the horse), fairly accurate lists of anatomical parts of the horse and of man have been preserved and transmitted, primarily through the exegetical Brāhmaṇa-texts. Filliozat's efforts at defining many of these parts have greatly advanced our understanding of the individual terms. Difficulties, however, still remain in the proper identification of many of the internal parts, which tend to be described by the native authorities in terms of a locality or as attached to a known organ. These enumerations provided the principal sources of anatomical knowledge until the time of the classical treatises (*saṁhitās*) of Āyurvedic medicine, when the visual inspection of the body by a type of dissection was introduced, perhaps from the West, into the traditional system of medical education.

Vedic medicine may be characterized essentially as a magico-religious system. Such a hackneyed definition implies more than it expresses. Space does not permit a complete discussion of magico-religious medicine and it is apparently opposite to empirical medicine. Causes of diseases are not attributed to physiological functions, but rather to external beings or forces of a demonic nature who enter the body of their victim and produce sickness. The removal of such malevolent entities usually involved an elaborate ritual, often drawing on aspects of the dominant local religion and nearly always necessitating spiritually potent and efficacious words, actions and devices. To some extent, the empirical medicine was also evident during Vedic time. It involved both observation and experience in order to determine the cause of disease and to effect an appropriate treatment.

The Vedic Indian's attitude toward disease, therefore, was dominated by the belief that evil spirits, demons and other malevolent forces invaded the body and caused their victims to exhibit a state of disease. These demons were often personified and deified, giving rise to an entire pantheon of gods of disease. The impetus for the attack may have come from a breach of a certain taboo, from a sin committed against the god or from witchcraft and sorcery. Injuries such as broken bones or wounds, however, were considered to be accidentally caused or the result of warfare. Other external diseases and afflictions were noticed to have been caused by noxious insects and vermin, often thought to be demonic in character.

The idea of health in a positive sense is wanting in Vedic medicine. Any notion of the concept is to be found in the negative or opposite of what was understood to be disease, or more specifically in the absence of particular disease-causing demons, of injuries and damages and of toxins.

As among most cultures of the world, an individual was considered to be healthy if his life-time was long, i.e., if he could repeatedly witness the rising sun, and if he showed complete recovery from illness. There are also indications that a wholesome body was associated with the intake of nutritious food.

The healing ritual always required the recitation of religious incantations or charms. An analysis of these verses illustrates certain apotropaic devices which included the use of sympathetic magic, of the rhetorical question, of onomatopoeic sounds, of the identifying name, of the esoteric word or phrase which, when properly uttered, focused the demon's attention on the healer, leading to its loss of grip and power. Disease-demons were often transferred from the patient to enemies or less desirable people, dispelled into the ground or carried away by birds to places where they could no longer be a menace to the community. Amulets or talismans (*maṇi*, literally 'jewel'), usually of vegetal origin, were ritually bound to drive out demons and to act as prophylactic measures in preventing further attacks. Fragrant plant substances were burnt to help expel the patient's demon, to protect him, and to make his environment pure and generally favourable for healing. Early morning (dawn), noon, and dusk (twilight) seem to have been the most auspicious times of the day to carry out healing rituals. Some rites were performed when certain stars were in a particular part of the heavens, suggesting that astrology may have played an important role in Vedic medicine.

In addition to the evidence of a systematic, classificatory way of thinking, the Vedic healers showed that they were familiar with some empirical procedures of healing. These therapeutic actions, however, are found in the context of the magico-religious rites, implying that their efficacy was inextricably connected with the magical or spiritual operation. The treatments worked because the proper words were recited, the correct actions performed and the right devices used.

Quite naturally these procedures are encountered most frequently in the treatment of external diseases and afflictions. For example, a form of surgery, utilizing a reed as a catheter, was performed to cure urine-retention; lancing and salt were used in the treatment of certain pustules; cauterization with caustic medicines and perhaps with fire was practised; sand and perhaps also reeds were applied to stop the flow of blood issuing from a wound and perhaps from the uterus; a resin was applied to wounds to prevent them from bleeding and to aid in the healing process; ointments and dyes were applied to the skin; a special plant was used which evidently promoted the growth of hair; and certain plants may also have been used in salves or poultices. Perhaps the most important empirical method of healing was the use of water as a type of hydrotherapy. It was employed for numerous ailments, both internal and external, suggesting that it was looked on as a significant therapeutic agent. The medicinal uses of water may well have evolved from the medical tradition of the Harappans.

Before examining and presenting in translations the most significant hymns which constitute the principal doctrinal remains of the Vedic phase of Indian medicine, we should have some idea of the Vedic medical lore in later centuries. In the earliest Āyurvedic treatises of Bhela, Caraka and Suśruta a reverence for Vedic medicine, as exemplified in the Atharva-veda, is advocated. In actual practice, however, a few of these early techniques seem to have survived. As an example, magico-religious utterances or *mantras,* which form the cornerstone of Vedic medicine, are found to have been used principally in five ways : 1. the treatment of swellings or tumors and wounds or sores (*śotha, vraṇa*); 2. the treatment of poison (*viṣa*); 3. the treatment of mental disorders (*unmatta, apasmāra*); 4. the treatment of fever (*jvara*); and 5. the collection and preparation of certain medicines. Parallels in Vedic medicine occur for each category. Often the similarities between the archaic and the Āyurvedic uses of *mantras* are remarkable. Vestiges of Vedic medicine are clearly represented by these five groups.

Agniveśa raised the point whether human beings are not suffering from the same diseases. What is the use of storing herbal medicines and different types of food to eradicate diseases? Atreya appreciated the point, but said that different diseases affect people. The reasons for such diseases are wind, water, place and time. Seasonal variation causes wind to blow hot or cold. Wind also carries dust and smoke. They are injurious to health. Contaminated water causes health hazards. Not only human beings but also animals, fish and birds avoid using it. Breeding centres for reptiles, flies, mosquitoes etc., are not safe places for habitation and storage of food grains. Seasonal changes such as summer, rains, winter, etc., also increase misery of living beings. All these contribute for the spread of disease. An environment free from all these extraneous causes is considered safe for healthy living. Timely check-up and administering proper medicine will help in curing diseases.

Agniveśa is curious to know the reasons for the spread of disorder in elements which cause havoc and destruction of living beings. Atreya reminds him of the Vedic tradition that any deviation from the path of Dharma by both the ruler and the ruled causes large-scale calamities. He elaborates on the meaning of अधर्म which is regarded as the main cause for spread of diseases and destruction. He reminds of *Satyayuga* when virtue guided the practice of Dharma and the result was that heavens had descended on this earth. People were free from fear, passion, jealousy, sorrow, disease, fatigue, stress, laziness, etc. All were happy and contented. Early part of *Kṛtayuga* was also very conducive to health, prosperity and progress. But the latter part of *Kṛtayuga* witnessed a rapid decline in values and people became pleasure-loving. They gave up hard work. They became greedy and selfish. In the *Tretāyuga* greed encouraged animosity resulting in group clashes due to frailties of the mind. The nature of the five elements also changed causing widespread havoc for the living beings. People lost their will power and became victims of *Vāta, Pitta* and *Kapha.* In *Kaliyuga* now, the disappearance of Dharma has resulted in untold miseries and suffering for living beings in the universe.[12]

The concept of the four *yugas* and the steady decline of values causing all sorts of maladies may not hold good in this scientific and technological age. Just as diseases are not common to all and they vary from person to person and place to place in accordance with seasonal variations. Similarly, the span of life is subject to be either short or long due to lack of discipline or a disciplined way of life. Lack of discipline causes अकालमृत्यु—untimely death—and a disciplined way of life ends in कालमृत्यु. Atreya explains this secret to Agniveśa in a rational and homely style :

'O Agniveśa! Listen to this. The axle of a chariot is well-tested and is of a fine quality. As time passes, the axle becomes weak and one day the chariot will break into pieces. In the same way, the body of a person with the passage of time becomes weak and one day his time comes. This is called कालमृत्यु.'[13]

The life span is broadly divided into three divisions—childhood, youth and old age. Suśruta has divided life span as बाल, मध्य and वृद्ध—Infancy and childhood, youth and the old age. बाल is divided into three divisions : क्षीरप (drinking milk only), क्षीरान्नदा (drinking milk and eating food) and the third is अन्नाद—only eating food. क्षीरप is one year from birth, क्षीरान्नदा is two years from birth and the rest is अन्नाद. The duration of मध्य or middle age is from sixteen to seventy years. Beyond seventy it is old age when the system starts decaying.[14] Age of a patient is a great factor to be kept in mind by the physician before prescribing any medicine and determining its dosage.

Medicines are also regarded as belonging to three types—one is based on divine elements दैवव्यपाश्रय; the second is based on युक्तिव्यपाश्रय—elements and intellect and the third is based on सत्त्वावजय—self-restraint. Medicine pertaining to divine elements is medicine by uttering *mantra*—मंत्र. Combination of food and medicine is called युक्तिव्यपाश्रय. Controlling of the mind is known as सत्त्वावजय.

Atreya makes a revelation to Agniveśa when he mentions the category of persons who are permanent patients. He says Brāhmaṇas, Government officers, courtezans and Vaiśyas always suffer from diseases. A Brāhmaṇa always is engaged in *Vedapāṭha* and does not take his food in proper time. He neglects his health and suffers from diseases. A government officer always engaged in his routine does not care for his health. Courtezans have to fulfil the demands of the rulers. *Vaiśya,* busy in his trade, gets stuck up to one place and has no time for maintaining his health.[15]

This detailed description throws light on the minutest aspects of the subjects covered in the ancient texts as the science of life—आयुर्वेद—in our country from the earliest times. Even today ancient treatises on Āyurveda like *Aṣṭāṅga Hṛdaya* and *Aṣṭānga Saṅgraha* are considered as source material in medicine by posterity for Vāgbhata's rich contribution to this science of life.

Madhavaka is considered as the clinical diagnostician in the 9th century A.D. Vrindā's contribution to Āyurvedic medicine is also worth noting. He belonged to the 10th century.

Salihotra of the 8th century B.C. is held in great respect as the father of Ancient Indian veterinary science. Treatment of human beings, of course, formed an important aspect of Indian medicine. But it is interesting to note that treatment of animals, birds, plants and trees was not neglected here.

Vṛkshāyurveda—वृक्षायुर्वेद—by Surapala deals with the treatment of plant diseases.

Mātaṅgalīla of Nārāyaṇa treats the subject of the diseases of elephants.

Aśvāyurveda of Gana and *Aśvachikitsā* by Jayadūta and Nakula are related to the treatment of horses :

Aśvāyurveda was an important branch of study and copious literature is found on this subject :

1. अश्ववैद्यक - जयदत्त
2. योगमंजरी - वर्धमान
3. अश्ववैद्यक - दीपकर
4. अश्ववैद्यक - अग्निपुराण
5. युक्तिकल्पतरु - भोज
6. अश्वायुर्वेद - वाग्भट

Someśvara is also credited with having written a book on treatment of Horse and Elephant diseases.[16]

हस्त्यायुर्वेद-गजायुर्वेद by पालकाप्यमुनि is another interesting book on diseases and treatment of elephants.

In ancient India, Gold, Silver, Copper and Iron were frequently used in medicines. Iron was called *Kṛṣṇāyasa* or the black metal; copper was called *Lohitāyasa* or the red-metal. *Harita* (Yellow) was the name given to gold and *Rajata* (white) was the name by which silver was known. Yajurveda makes references to these metals as they were used for the fulfilment of sacrifices.[17] According to D.D. Mehta, "A regular science of mercury was developed as a branch of chemistry in ancient India. Iron and mercury are mentioned as aphrodisiacs and tonics by Varāhamihira (587 A.D.). There were several preparations of iron, copper, mercury, and other metals which were utilized in medicine."[18] *Rasa* meant mercury in the oldest Āyurvedic literature. Vātsyāyana's *Kāmasūtra* refers to sixty-four *kalās*, or arts,[19] that were practised by Indians of his time. Among them are mentioned the testing of gold and gems, the differentiating of gems according to their weight, hardness, lustre, transparency and colour, fusibility, especially when heated in combination with the alkalis, etc. As we can see from the above, subjects concerning Āyurveda have been found scattered in various literary works. King Someśvara has rendered great service to us by explaining these various subjects in a single monumental encyclopaedic work Rāja Mānasollāsa.

Reason of Diseases

Man does not live in an absolutely germ-free atmosphere. The only thing that can be done safely is to keep the tissues of the body unreceptive towards these germs. Once the human body is affected, the tissues should be so conditioned by drugs and diet and other regimens that these germs or bacteria, by whatsoever names they may be called, will find the atmosphere hostile towards their survival, multiplication and growth.

In the Rāja Mānasollāsa, Someśvara says that the change of normal condition is due to food and the bad actions of a man.[20] He explains how *doṣas* affect the human body. *Sāma* (undigested food) is the creator of the *doṣas*, and then it disturbs the *Jaṭharāgni*. This *Jaṭharāgni* spreads in the human body. This is called fever or *Jvara*. This *Jvara* is the king of all the diseases.[21] Further, it results into many varieties of diseases. In respect of each disease, whether named or unnamed, Someśvara says that the following points need careful attention.

Nidāna or Causative Factors

These causative factors are further divided into the following four categories : *Sannikṛṣṭa* or those which produce disease quite early, *Viprakṛṣṭa* or those having delayed effects in producing a disease, *Vyabhicārī* or those that are not strong enough to cause a disease and *Prādhānika* or those having instantaneous effects in producing the disease, viz., strong poisons. The causative factors can further be divided into two groups, namely, exogenous and endogenous. Various types of dust, regimens and the effects of seasons are the exogenous factors. Vitiation of *Doṣas (Vāta, Pitta* and *Kapha)* or *Prakṛtis* and *Dhātus* are the endogenous factors to cause a disease.

Pūrvarūpa or Premonitory symptoms

These premonitory symptoms are of two types, viz., general and specific. Some of the premonitory symptoms only indicate the nature of the disease going to be manifested in general.

Rūpa or Manifested signs and symptoms

When the disease is fully manifested, certain signs and symptoms appear. In the Āyurvedic texts, signs and symptoms of each of these diseases are described in detail. Rāja Mānasollāsa explains वैद्यशास्त्रानुसारेण कारयेत् तत्प्रतिक्रियाम्। (1-19-143), These are indicative of the stage of the disease and of the *Doṣas*,

Dhātus, Agnis, as well as *Śrotas* involved in the manifestation of the disease. They also indicate the prognosis of the disease. On the basis of these signs and symptoms, therapies, diet and regimens are prescribed for the patient.

Upaśya or Exploratory therapy

Sometimes, the causative factor, premonitory symptoms and actual symptoms of the disease, do not well indicate the nature of the disease. A physician in such conditions, resorts to some exploratory therapy to ascertain correctly the nature of the disease. These are the common characteristics of all the Āyurvedic works. But Rāja Mānasollāsa gives some more information for a careful examination of the disease. Someśvara gives importance to the time and place, and also *Sātmya Prakṛti.* It means the strength of the patient. Further, it tells that a physician should know the *Svarūpa* or features of a disease, and *Lakṣaṇa* i.e., symptoms or distinctive characteristics of the disease and so on.

Jvara or Fever

Jvara or fever occupies the first place among physical ailments. So Someśvara's Rāja Mānasollāsa describes it first and tells that *Jvara* or fever is the king of all diseases. *Mādhavanidānam* [माधवनिदानम् of Sri Mādhavācar, Chaukhambha Sanskrit Sansthan, Varanasi, 1981] says that—Rudra was creator of *Jvara* and it is in eight parts.

दक्षापमानसंक्रुद्धरुद्रनिःश्वाससंभवः।
ज्वरोऽष्टधा पृथग्द्वन्द्वसंघातागन्तुजः स्मृतः॥ 2.1

Carakasaṁhitā says[22] that there are eight types of *Jvara.* In Rāja Mānasollāsa it has no definite number. Someśvara divides on the basis of *doṣas,* viz., *Vātapitta Jvara,*[23] *Vāta-jvara,*[24] and so on (1.19.160-196). *Carakasaṁhitā* further states the causative factors of the fever.[25] The factors responsible for the causation of fever in human beings are *Vāta, Pitta, Kapha, Vātapitta,*

Vātakapha, Pittakapha, Vātapittakapha. There is the other extrinsic factor also. Only the immediate causes of fever are mentioned here. These causes are concerned with the fever of human beings only. Those of the other animals like horses, elephants, cows and birds may be different.

Someśvara's Rāja Mānasollāsa gives the names of animals' fever, birds' fever, the fever of plants and so on.[26] Fever caused by all these categories has one thing in common, that is, pain precedes the occurrence of fever in all such cases. Hence, they are treated as of one type in the eight-fold classification of *Jvara.* Hence, Someśvara says, "there is only one type of *Jvara,* but it has many names."

Treatment of Fever

During the stage of *Pūrvarūpa* (premonitory symptoms) or in the primary stage of *Jvara,* intake of light food or fasting is useful, because *āmāśaya* (stomach including small intestine) is the site of origin of this disease. There is no contradiction in these statements because the intake of light diet is only a form of *Laṅghana* and produces lightness in the body.[27] Further, in *vātika* type of *Jvara,* complete fasting is prohibited as it aggravates *Vāta* taking part in the pathogenesis of the disease. In such a condition, intake of light diet is prescribed. Normally, even light diet should aggravate *vāta*, but it does not do so in a patient suffering from *Jvara* because the site of origin of disease in *āmāśaya* and all aggravated *doṣas* residing here including *vāta* are corrected by the intake of light diet.

In the Rāja Mānasollāsa, Someśvara discusses the preparation of medicines or *Kaṣāyas* and their utility for fever and other diseases. In all the types of chronic fever and other diseases, intake of ghee is beneficial,[28] because it acts both against the diseases as well as the *doṣas* involved. "As people spray water over a house set on fire, so also ghee should be used with a view to alleviate chronic fever and other diseases.[29] *Vāta* is alleviated due to latter's unctuousness, *Pitta* due to coldness and even *Kapha* due to suitable method of preparation.

Rāja Mānasollāsa further discusses all types of *Jvara*, and many varieties of medicines. *Raktapitta*[30] (a disease characterised by bleeding from various parts of the body), is caused by the heat of *Jvara*. This *Raktapitta* is not the combination of *rakta* (blood) and *pitta*. It is only a pathological state of *pitta*. This disease manifests itself in two ways, either through upper tracks or through the lower tracks. In a patient having the dominance of *Kapha* in his body, the disease manifests itself in blood coming out through the upper tracks, viz., ear, nose, eyes and mouth. In a patient whose body is dominated by *Vāta*, the disease manifests itself in blood coming out through the lower tracks, viz., the urethra and anus. In a patient whose body is dominated by both *Kapha* and *Vāta*, the disease manifests itself through both the tracks mentioned above. The first type of *Rakta-pitta*, where the upper tracks are afflicted, is curable because of its amenability to purgation therapy and also because varieties of drugs are available for the treatment of this condition. The second type of *Raktapitta* is called by Someśvara as *Yāpya*. *Yāpya* type of *Rakta-pitta*, where the lower tracks are afflicted, is palliable because of its amenability to emetic therapy and also because of the limited varieties of drugs available for its treatment. The third type where both the upper and lower tracks are afflicted is incurable because it is neither amenable to purgation nor to emetic therapy and no medicine is suitable for the treatment of this condition. Hence Someśvara's advice is, "the enlightened physician should not take incurable patient in hand. The palliable patient should be maintained with appropriate therapy. The curable one should be treated carefully with proper medicine leading to cure."[31] Someśvara describes the *Kaṣāya* which is meant to control the *Rakta-pitta*.[32]

After dealing with fever, its characteristic features, and remedies, Someśvara continues to explain on similar lines, many other diseases. The details of these are given below.

1. *Kṣaya* : Someśvara says that highly polluted air enters the body and increases *Pitta* and *Kapha*. Then it enters the joints of the body. Thus *Kṣaya* is caused. According to him, the patient of this disease should swallow the *Cūrṇa of Rāsnā, Tila* and *Balā* mixed with ghee, *Yastikī* (Jeṣṭhamadhū) and Utpala to get cured from this disease.[33]

2. *Chardi-roga* (Vomitting) : Someśvara has mentioned that this disease is caused by consuming food which is not at all suited for one's health.[34] According to him this disease can be remedied by making the patient drink the mixture of honey, *Kaṣāya,* made from the budding leaves of *Jamboo, Cūta, Balā, Uśīra, Vaṭa* and *Śuṅga.*[35]

3. *Madātyaya, Moha, Bhrama Tandrā* and *Pralāpa.*[36] Someśvara says that these are caused by excessive and faulty drinking of wine. *Madātyaya* lasts for about five to seven days. If it lasts for more days than this, it is to be understood that it is some other disease.[37]

Someśvara has said that this disease can be remedied by eating '*Saktupiṣṭa*' with the mutton extract of goat, deer, rabbit, Tittira and Lāva birds or by drinking sweet *Pānaka* or ghee.[38] Someśvara says that these are the best remedies to cure such diseases.

4. *Arśas* : He says that this is a disease caused by the protrusions (*Aṅkura*) appearing in the region of *Gudadvāra* (Anus) and intestine (*Āntrāvali*) as a result of prolonged *maladhāraṇa* (constipation).[39] Someśvara has suggested that this disease can be remedied by applying the paste formed by the mixture of *Śṛṅgī, Haritakī, Kuṣṭa, Bhallātaka* fruits, and *Tuthya* (Blue-vitriol) at the region of *Gudadvāra.*[40] Further, he has suggested that applying the paste formed by *Mūla,* (Amarphophallus), *Śighrubīja* (Drumstick seed), *Niṁba* (Neem) and *Asvatha* leaves, *Bilva*-fruits, *akroda* root (or *Pīlumūla*) and *Rāmaṭha* at the *Gudadvāra* eradicates the *Aṅkuras* (Protrusions).[41]

5. *Atisāra* : Someśvara says that this is due to over-drinking

of water. He has hinted at the remedies for the three types of this disease.

Remedies

In the Rāja Mānasollāsa, the author states about *Ratnaparīkṣā* (2.4. 530-536). Gems, were considered helpful in medicines. Someśvara tells about the origin of gems, or *Maṇis*. 'The place of origin of *Padmarāgamaṇi* is Siṁhaḷa. Similarly, *Kuruvinda-maṇi* is found in Kālapura, and *Saugandhamaṇi* is obtained in Andhra.[42] Further, Someśvara tells that *Padmaragamaṇi* is the best in all the *maṇis* or gems. The place of origin of the *Indranīlamaṇi* is Siṁhaḷadvīpa. It has four varieties, namely, White, Red, Yellow, and Black (2.4. 492-493). Next, the author tells about its characteristics, merits, demerits and so on (2.4. 494-506). The place of origin of *Marakatamaṇi* is Turkasthāna. It has seven demerits, five merits and eight shades (2.4. 507-508). The origin of *Sphaṭikamaṇi* is the Himalaya, Siṁhaḷa, Vindhya, and the bank of Tāpi river. Herein the main divisions are two, namely *Sūryakānta* and *Candrakānta* (2.4. 520). Further, Someśvara says, "*Candrakāntamaṇi* is not available in this Kaliyuga." Then he describes *Puṣparāga, Vaiḍūrya, Gomedha* and *Vidruma*. Further, Someśvara gives the characteristics of the *maṇis* or gems. A good gem should be put into milk. If the milk changes its colour and becomes blue, the gem is called *Indranīla*. It is loved by God Śanaiścara'.[43] The gems have their own characteristics, first of all heaviness, second spotlessness, third lustre or rediance and fourth inflexibility or hardness. These are the common characteristics.[44] The uses of gems are—*Indranīlamaṇi* gives wealth, life, strength, and fame.[45] The *Marakatamaṇi* is used to counteract poison.[46]

1. *Āmātisāra* : *Kṣāya* of the *cūrṇas* of *Rāmaṭha*, or *Nāgara, Mustā, Ghurṇavallabha*, should be taken along with food to promote digestion of food.[47]

2. *Pakvātisāra* : The mixture of honey, with boiled *Jambūpallava, Dhātakī Jīraka, Cūtabīja, Mahāvṛkṣatvaca, Bilva, Aranāla, Gokaṅṭa, Pancāṅgula* and *Yava* is the medicine for this disease.[48]

3. *Raktātisāra* : The *Kaṣāya* of the mixture of *Viṣā, Kuṭajabīja, Mustā, Vālaka* and *Bilva* is the medicine for this disease.[49]

Further, Someśvara has stated that a person who does not take hygienic food while suffering from *Atisāraroga,* suffers from a disease called *Grahaṇīroga.* He has said that *Grahaṇīroga* can be remedied by taking the *Kaṣāya* of *Śuṇṭhi, Ativiṣā Mustā*, and also *Guḍūci.*

Regarding *Mūtrakṛchra,* Someśvara says that it starts pain in the joints of the body especially in *Mehana* (Urinary track). He has mentioned the remedies for the *Mūtrakṛchra* disease. According to him this disease can be remedied by making the patient drink *Kaṣāya* made from *Urabūka, Balā, Bilva,* two *Pancamūla (Laghu Pancamūla* and *Bṛhat Pancamūla), Yavā, Punarnavā, Bhīrumūla, Kulattha, Badara, Matsyākṣa, Matsyābheda* and mixed with ghee as well as oil. The fat of a hog and bear mixed with fine *lavaṇas (Samudra, Saindhava, Bīdala, Pāde* and *Kācala lavaṇa)*[50] should be added to the *Kaṣāya.* Someśvara says that these are the best remedies to cure such diseases.

Thus, we find that Someśvara has shown keen interest in the eradication of various diseases. This also exhibits his deep knowledge regarding the use of various medicinal plants and herbs, though he was a king.

In the light of all these discussions, it appears to be appropriate for Someśvara to express his opinion regarding the medicines. Someśvara says, medicines should not be—

1. देशविरुद्ध in antagonism to climate and soil.
2. कालविरुद्ध in antagonism to season.

3.	अग्निविरुद्ध	in antagonism to digestive capacity of juices.
4.	सात्म्यासात्म्य	in antagonism to the constitution and diathesis of the patient.
5.	संस्कारविरुद्ध	in antagonism to the mode of preparation.
6.	रसविरुद्ध वीर्यविरुद्ध	incompatible pharmacologically.
7.	कोष्टविरुद्ध	detrimental to the condition of the digestive organs, in relation to their susceptibility.
8.	अवस्थाविरुद्ध	affecting the general condition of the patient with reference to the time of administration.
9.	क्रमविरुद्ध	such as would disturb the methods of arrangement in the administration of drugs.
10.	(परिहार/उपचार) –विरुद्ध	inconsistent with the nature of the course prescribed.
11.	पाकविरुद्ध	violating the rules of the preparation of drugs.
12.	संयोगविरुद्ध	incompatible, either chemically or physically.
13.	हृद्विरुद्ध	such as would disturb the mental attitude, e.g., those creating aversion towards certain drugs.
14.	संपद्विरुद्ध	deficient in pharmacological or nutritional properties.
15.	विधिविरुद्ध	such as would affect the actual way or procedure in which food is taken.

The methods of diagnosis adopted by the Āyurvedists, like

those of the methods adopted in the Western system of medicine, depend upon the close observation of the patient, his mental and bodily conditions, environments and such factors are necessary to be understood to trace the origin and progress of the disease. In this connection Vāgbhaṭa says :

तस्माद्विकारप्रकृतीरधिष्ठानान्तराणि च।
बुद्ध्वा हेतुविशेषांश्च शीघ्रं कुर्यादुपक्रमम्।।
दूष्यं देशं बलं कालमनल प्रकृतिं वयः
सत्त्वं सात्म्यं तथाऽऽहारमवस्थाश्च पृथग्विधा।।
सूक्ष्मसूक्ष्माः समीक्ष्यैषां दोषौषधनिरूपणे।
यो वर्तते चिकित्सायां न स स्खलति जातुचित्।

–(अ.हृ.सू.अ. 12.66-68)

The physician should first ascertain the nature of the disease, the derangement caused in it by the *doṣas,* the situations or the organs where the derangement is manifested and the causes which are responsible for this derangement, and then begin to treat the disease. He who, during the examination of the patient, considers the conditions of the *dhātus* and the *malas,* the place of his residence, his strength and power of tolerance, the season of the ailment in question, the power of digestion, constitution and diathesis, the age, the mental state, the habits (likings) and idiosyncrasies, the food usually taken and other minute items related to the patient, and then arrives at a diagnosis and commences treatment, will never commit any mistake.

From this, it will be clear that the foundations of rational therapeutics are almost the same in both the ancient and the modern systems of medicine. In Āyurveda, *Satva, Sātmya, Doṣa* and *Dooṣya* have been looked upon with greater regard than in modern medicine. We have seen that the concept of the theory of 'Cause and Effect' has received greater importance not only from the evolutionary point of view, but also from the standpoint of practical medicine. The *Tridoṣa* theory, which is made to confirm the *Pañca-bhautika* conception, is throughout used as the basis for the investigation of disease and therapeutics.

In pursuance of the definition of 'Life', Mind, the other side of the human constitution, has, from the earliest times, been rightly considered as a possible factor in the causation of disease. *Rajas* and *Tamas* are stated to be the causes of mental disturbance-disorder. Psycho-therapeutics had, therefore, long been in vogue in India. In modern times too, the significance of psychology and its relation to medicine has been well recognised. In treatment, one has, therefore, to dive into the subconscious regions of the mind, in order to trace the course of the mental disorders. Consciousness (जागृति) is not an essential condition for the mental processes. Significant changes may go on in the mind of a person without his/her being conscious of them. It is in this subconscious region that the root causes of mental disorders lie.

Vāgbhaṭa insists on the necessity of the consideration of *Satva* along with *Sātmya*, *Doṣa* and *Dooṣya*. Here *Satva* points to the state of the mind. *Sātmya* to the susceptibilities, peculiarities and tendencies, *Doṣa* to the pathogenic factors and *Dooṣya* to the changes in the seven primary tissues *(Sapta-dhātus)*.

The appearance of disease (आमय), as Āyurvedists have repeatedly stated, first takes place in the *Ādya-dhātu* owing to the irregularities of food and drink, rest, exercise, variations in living etc. Unless the *rasa* is contaminated or the *dhātus* contained in the *rasa* are disturbed by अयोग, अतियोग or मिथ्यायोग, no disease can come into existence. This variation first manifests itself in the form of वृद्धि or क्षय in the सूक्ष्मावयवs of the *dhātus* concerned. The principle that underlies these processes has been enunciated as—

वृद्धिः समानैः सर्वेषां विपरीतैः विपर्ययः ।

–(अ.हृ.सू. 1.3)

The *dhātus* of the body after getting nourishment from the different articles of food naturally assume the corresponding properties of the latter. There are, as Caraka points out, तत्रेमे

शरीरधातुगुणाः संख्यासामर्थ्यकरास्तद्यथा-गुरुलघुशीतोष्णम्।।-(चरकसंहिता-शा० 6.10)

An excess or deficiency of these properties in the first place gives rise to दोषदुष्टि (diseased processes) and secondly to धातुदुष्टि (diseased structures) and स्थानदुष्टि (diseased organs). These three represent the pathology, morbid anatomy, and organic derangements, respectively, Caraka says,

कार्ययोनिर्धातुवैषम्यं, तस्य लक्षणं विकारागमः।।

-(चरकसंहिता-वि० 8.14)

Nidāna-Pañcaka

In Āyurveda, the methods of investigation of diseases are usually described under the following five heads :

(a) निदान (*Nidāna*), (b) पूर्वरूप (*Pūrva-rūpa*), (c) रूप (*Rūpa*), (d) उपशय (*Upaśaya*) and (e) संप्राप्ति (*Samprāpti*).

These are known as "निदानपंचक" where *Nidāna* means "रोगनिश्चय."

(a) ***Nidāna*** **:** Means the 'root-cause of the disease' and may be बाह्य (external), आभ्यंतर (internal), विप्रकृष्ट (remote), सन्निकृष्ट (immediate and hence exciting), प्रधानिक (primary), or व्यभिचारि (minor).

Nidāna is brought about by—

1. असात्म्येंद्रियार्थसंयोग—incompatible correlation of the senses with their objects, i.e., transgression of the power of tolerance; e.g., exposure to cold, causing nasal or pulmonary catarrh.
2. प्रज्ञापराध—Indiscretion in behaviour and irregularity in life,
3. External influences such as seasonal and climatic factors.

(b) ***Pūrvarūpa*** **:** Is suggestive of premonitory symptoms. The symptoms only suggest that some internal derangement has been started and that toxins are making their way towards the tissue-cells : दोषदूष्यसंमूर्च्छनावस्था. The infection is still undeveloped and does not show any characteristics of a particular दोष (disease) : लिंगमव्यक्तमल्पत्वात् व्याधीनाम. It is a precursor of future trouble.

(c) ***Rūpa*** **:** When the दोष develops there is a clear manifestation of subjective symptoms and physical signs. These signs and symptoms go by the names : रूप, लिंग, लक्षण, आकृति, संस्थान.

(d) ***Upaśaya*** **:** Caraka explains *'Upaśaya'* as सात्म्ययार्थो हि उपशयार्थ: in the eleventh chapter of *Sootrasthāna* and defines सात्म्य *(Sātmya)* in the eighth chapter of *Vimanasthāna* as 'सात्म्यं नाम तद्यत्सातत्येनोपसेव्यमानमुपशेते'. *Sātmya* is thus that property which, owing to a habitual use, develops adaptability. So, if a certain property in an article brings relief to a patient by removing the disturbing factor, it is said to be an *Upāśaya* of that derangement. सुखानुबंधो यो हेतुर्व्याध्यादिविपरीतक: (Sudant-Sen, Commentary on *Mādhava-Nidāna*). This is just like tracing the disease (cause) from the effect. In other words, it is an art—a device of diagnosing by "applied therapeutics". Caraka advises this method of diagnosis when the दोष is अव्यक्त; for he says गूढलिंगं व्याधिसुपशयानुपशयाभ्याम् परीक्षेत ।।–(चरकसंहिता–वि० 4.15)

(e) ***Samprāpti*** **:** Means the knowledge of the way in which a certain disease develops. By knowing the *Samprāpti*, almost all the circumstances related to the development of a disease, whether arising from intrinsic or incidental causes, can be estimated.

The main features of *Samprāpti* are described as संख्या विकल्प प्राधान्य बल काल विशेषत:–माधव निदान.

1. संख्या (*Samkhyā*) : The number of varieties or types in which diseases manifest themselves. This is, of course,

only a general statement and hence does not give any idea of the particulars.

2. विकल्प (*Vikalpa*) : दोषणामंशांशकल्पना. This gives a correct idea of the direction in which the different दोषs (toxins) have developed. This is eventually of great value in 'Treatment'.
3. प्राधान्य (*Prādhānya*) : Nature of the disease as to whether it is primary or secondary.
4. बल (*Bala*) : Severity or otherwise : (उत्तन—*Uttana* or गम्भीर—*Gambhīra*).
5. काल (*Kāla*) : Season, whether favourable or otherwise.

Next, the morbid phenomena which are ascertained by studying the क्रियाकाल (*Kriyākāla*) in *Samprāpti* are thus mentioned :

(i) संचय *(Sañcaya)* : means the Accumulation of दोषs.

(ii) प्रकोप *(Prakopa)* : means Excitation.

(iii) प्रसर *(Prasara)* : means Extension of lesion.

(iv) स्थानसंश्रय *(Sthānasamśraya)* : means Location of the affection.

(v) व्यक्ति *(Vyakti)* : manifestation of symptoms.

(vi) भेद *(Bheda)* : means variation in the spread of the disease.

It is thus clear that all the details of 'Pathology' are taken into consideration by the Āyurvedists in following these methods of diagnosis. Clinical descriptions of symptoms caused by pathological derangements in the दोषs and धातुs are given by Suśruta in the fifteenth chapter of *Sūtrasthāna* and by Vāgbhaṭa in the eleventh chapter of *Sūtrasthāna*.

In surgical pathology, naked-eye appearances characteristic of दोषs are minutely described in terms such as वर्ण, छाया, राग, दाह,

पाक, कंडू, तोद, शोथ, कोथ etc. For the symptoms and pathological manifestations, the reader should refer to the fifteenth chapter of Vāgbhaṭa's *Nidānasthāna* wherein detailed description of वातविकार *(Vātavikāra)* in the different आशयs *(Āśayas)*, धातुs *(Dhātus)* and स्रोतस् *(Srotas)* is given. Similarly, the derangements caused by *Pitta* and *Kapha* when they attack the सप्तधातुs (*Saptadhātus*) and the resultant symptoms are given in the nineteenth chapter of *Sootrasthāna* of Vāgbhaṭa's *Aṣṭāngasangraha.* Both these deserve to be thoroughly mastered for a thorough understanding of the real part played by the दोषs in their vitiated condition in respect of their influence on the body-tissues.

The pathology of निज and आगंतुकरोगs is described accordingly as they arise from intrinsic (धातुवैषम्य) and incidental (आगंतुक) causes respectively. Āyurvedists hold that even these आगंतुकदोषs, such as bacteria, have a constitution of their own which can be described in *Tridoṣa* terminology. These organisms have, after all, a material body which carry with them a type of *Pañca-bhautika* constitution. They grow under particular favourable conditions and die when the environment becomes unfavourable. The internal जंतुs are the resultant products of the *Tridoṣās,* while the external have their origin in the environment. In treatment, importance is given to both types, as they are likely to transgress their limits and encroach upon each other. Caraka has put this beautifully in the following words : आगंतुरन्वेति निजंविकारं निजस्तथा गंतुमपिप्रवृद्धः।।-(चरकसंहिता-सूत्रस्थान 20.18)

आगंतु (रोग) is defined by him in the next chapter.[51]

In *Āgantu* diseases, affliction is the first occurrence, and this is, in course of time, followed by derangement of the three *doṣas.* In निजविकार, *Vāta, Pitta* and *Kapha* are first deranged by some internal pathogenic cause, and then the symptoms (like pain) follow.

In the opinion of the Āyurvedists, the internal bacteria are only the result of failure in equilibrium in the body-constitution caused by chemical products of bad digestion. The chief reason why the ancient physicians do not totally depend upon the bacterial theory is, because of the non-applicability of that theory in all diseases and in all individuals. They, therefore, while reserving the germ theory, its own place in treatment, are not ready to assign to it an invariable position in the causation of disease. In short, the origin and cause of disease suggested in Āyurveda is placed on a broader basis.

According to Caraka,[52] diseases take place when toxins, singly or collectively, affect the lymphatics, blood vessels and the nerves in a person who takes insalutary food and has no control over his mind.

On studying the methods of *Roga-parīkṣā* till now gone over, one should be able to estimate the extent of the virulence of the *doṣas* or the disease itself. But there is another side of medical examination which is very important, and which, if neglected, would make all attempts of treatment useless. And this is 'आयुपरीक्षा', which means an approximate estimation of the state of natural resistance in an individual, both in normal as well as in the impaired conditions of health. It involves the investigation of various factors about the patient viz., those connected with his nature, temperament, constitution, hereditary influences, habit, environments, etc. (For particulars vide Caraka, *Vimāna,* Ch. 8). These undoubtedly throw a flood of light on the prognosis of the case and enable the physician to choose remedies of a definite potency. Caraka has given detailed description about the methods of understanding the personal constitution of the patient in the first chapter वर्णस्वरीय of इंद्रियस्थान. This part of investigation is often neglected both by students and *vaidyas* and it will be no exaggeration to say that no method of treatment would be complete and successful without a knowledge of personal vitality and power of resistance of a patient. असात्म्येन्द्रियार्थसंयोग. The first condition mentioned in the array of etiological factors points to the natural resistance of an individual to disease. In fact, the first three stages, चय, प्रकोप and प्रसार, in the development of the disease, are directly connected with the personal resistance of the patient. The question of tempering the virulence or checking the progress of the disease depends upon a clear understanding of the elementary factors in *Samprāpti.* The significance of this, especially in treatment, is well expressed by Vāgbhaṭa.[53]

An attempt should always be made to check the accumulation of *doṣas*; but when the toxins are already there, treatment should be so adopted, whether by means of diet or medicines, that it does not provoke further complications. When all the three *doṣas* are affected, one should aim at removing the affection which is more harmful or more advanced.

The credit of bringing these elementary principles of pathology really falls to the share of ancient Āyurvedists. Except through the agency of *Tridoṣa* theory or some other, which is akin to it, it is not possible to understand the *samcaya* stage in the *samprāpti* of a disease. There is no doubt that imagination has to be stretched and inferences drawn upon probabilities and possibilities. Even in laboratory work much of imagination, discrimination and reasoning are required to arrive at conclusions. In research work, it is often found that theory and practice scarcely differ. The first directs the second, while the second confirms the truth of the first, Caraka expresses the same idea in the following words : प्रत्यक्षं तु खालु तत्, यत् स्वयमिन्द्रियैर्मनसा चोपलभ्यते ।।-(चरकसंहिता-वि० 4.5)

This sort of thought-sequence is necessary to understand the दोषदूष्यसंमूर्च्छनावस्था—the basis of *samacaya* and to trace its development further and correlate the particular *doṣa* with the particular symptoms.

आयु:परीक्षा and व्याधि परीक्षा Treatment

It must first be noted that the unique feature of Āyurvedic

treatment rests on the consideration not only of आयुपरीक्षा and व्याधिपरीक्षा, but also on the means and methods of application of medicines. Caraka, at the very beginning of *Sūtrasthānās,* divides the whole subject of Āyurveda into two parts : 1. हेतुलिंगाऔषधज्ञानम् and 2. स्वस्थातुरपरायणम्. हेतु and लिंग, which embrace etiology, symptomatology and pathology. Some of the details of औषध will be treated in the following portion.

स्वस्थवृत्त, i.e., attention to the personal well-being, is looked upon with equal importance in Āyurveda along with *Roga-Chikitsā.* It forms part of the subject of medicine and is not treated as a different subject as in western system. स्वास्थ्य is defined as दोषसाम्यमरोगता also as Caraka[54] has referred.

'Health' is defined as that condition of the body when the three *doṣas* of a person are in equipoise, his power of digestion is normal, the *dhātus* and *malas* are in proper order, he is cheerful, his mind is undisturbed and his sensory organs are normal.

Equilibrium in the three *doṣas*-the symbolic expressions of the three important stages of the body, is a necessary factor for the maintenance of health. The words समाग्नि and प्रसन्नात्मेंद्रियमना: are significant. In common practice, these do not receive so much attention as they deserve. In the case of treatment, Āyurvedists have given importance to प्रकृतिस्थापन and not restricted themselves to the cure of symptoms alone. If there is any speciality in the technique of treatment, it is this devotion of attention to the restoration of health. *Doṣa-Sāmya* constitutes the first consideration in treatment. This sententious word carries with it a world of meaning. For, the effective character of all the numerous forms of treatment, finds a place in the realization of *Doṣa-Sāmya.* Caraka says,[55] maintenance of equilibrium in the three *dhātus* is the primary object intended in treatment; and maintenance of hygiene (स्वास्थ्य) also requires the same precaution, viz., *Dhātu-Sāmya.*

In order to attain these ends, Āyurvedists proposed the following methods of treatment. These are classified into two main groups :

1. संतर्पण or बृंहण. 2. अपतर्पण or लंघन. पार्थिव and आप्यद्रव्यs characterise the former, and आग्नेय, वायव्य and आकाशीय the latter. लंघन again consists of two forms, viz., शोधन and शमन. Of these, शोधन can be accomplished by (a) वमन, (b) विरेचन, (c) शिरोविरेचन, (d) बस्ति and (e) अस्रविमोचन and शमन can be accomplished by (a) पाचन, (b) दीपन, (c) क्षूत् (अन्नवर्जन) (d) तृट् (उदकवर्जन), (e) व्यायाम (f) आतप and (g) मरुत्.

The whole list comprises of the following forms :

1. बृंहण—Tonics.
2. स्नेहन—Protectives, Emollients and Demulcents.
3. स्तंभन—Astringents.
4. वमन—Emetics.
5. शोधन—Purgatives and Diuretics.
6. नस्य—Sternutatories.
7. बस्ति—Enema and Douchings.
8. अस्रविमोचन—Blood-letting.
9. शोधन—Diaphoretics.
10. शोषण—Absorbents.
11. पाचन—Digestives and Carminatives.
12. दीपन—Stimulants; Respiratory, Cardiac, Nerve and Gastro-intestinal.
13. क्षुत्—Fasting.
14. तृट्—Restriction of water (thirst).
15. व्यायाम—Exercise.
16. आतप—Fomentation.
17. मरुत्—Ventilation.

The modes of therapeutic action included in these different forms of treatment fall under six heads :

1. हेतुविपरीत	corresponds to Rational.
2. व्याधिविपरीत	corresponds to Symptomatic.
3. हेतुव्याधिविपरीत	corresponds to Rational and Symptomatic.
4. हेतुतदर्थकारी	These involve the
5. व्याधितदर्थकारी	Principle 'Similia similibus'
6. हेतुव्याधितदर्थकारी	'curanteur.'

The first three are clear enough and need no explanation. The remaining three form the basic principles of homeopathy, where medicines which create the same condition as the disease, are used.

In Āyurveda and modern medicine, the first three lines of treatment are chiefly used. In the former हेतुविपरीतचिकित्सा receives the closest attention, as *Dhātus-Vaishamya* whether brought on by *Nija* or *Āgantuka* causes is the chief object for attack. Undoubtedly this subjective view of the Āyurvedists has a greater advantage over the objective methods of व्याधिविपरीत-चिकित्सा. व्याधि is, after all, a symptom and may be produced by a number of causes. For instance, headache may be caused by derangement in any one of the three *doṣas*. The right application of medicine would be to remove the cause first as it automatically removes the diseases also. In the treatment of acute diseases, such as fever, this method is greatly useful. In chronic diseases, as there is a jumble of symptoms brought on by व्याधिसंकर, any one of the two or both have to be used. There are, again, some diseases where the primary symptoms are not detected; in such cases, symptoms, which are after all the manifestations of the cause, require to be treated. Suśruta explains this as, in cases where there are sequels and complications great discretion has to be used in choosing the line of treatment. One has to meet the circumstances of the case and treat it accordingly. Because, when the complication is severe and intolerable, it requires to be necessarily treated first. The instructions of Vāgbhaṭa are very clear on this point (Vide Chapter 12 and 13 of *Sūtrasthāna).* Palliative and symptomatic lines have their own place in treatment and so cannot be neglected. Similarly, a heroic line of treatment should not be adopted without a consideration of all the causative factors and their progress in the evolution of all the stages of disease. For, a natural elimination of toxins is always in operation on the part of the organism, and any attempt to disturb it, is bound to be harmful.

Clinical Examination

The clinical examination in Āyurveda is conducted with the knowledge given by I. *Pratyakṣa.* II. *Anumāna.* III. *Āptvacana.*

I. प्रत्यक्ष (पंचभि:श्रोत्रादिभि:प्रश्नेन च).

II. अनुमान.

III. आप्तवचन.

I. *Pratyakṣa-Parīkṣā* (प्रत्यक्षपरीक्षा) includes examination by the five senses and by asking direct questions to the patient or to his relatives.

The following are the five senses used for *Pratyakṣa-Parīkṣā.*

(a) श्रोत्रेंद्रिय ग्राह्य	By hearing sounds, noises etc., and by marking the voice.
(b) स्पर्शनेंद्रिय ग्राह्य	By touching, feeling and manipulating with hand.
(c) चक्षुरिंद्रिय ग्राह्य	By seeing the various parts and noting the changes therein.
(d) रसनेंद्रिय ग्राह्य	(1) By judging the taste of the discharges, secretions and excretions as felt by insects such

as ants, flies, etc., and (2) by inquiry into the nature of the tongue and taste in the mouth.

(e) घ्राणेंद्रिय ग्राह्य — By smelling the discharges, excretions and breath.

Modern books contain detailed information on this most important subject and the students do well by referring to such books. The methods given in Āyurveda are exactly analogus to inspection, percussion, auscultation and mensuration as understood in modern literature. Since the advent of the thermometer, the stethoscope, the microscope and various other instruments for examining the eyes, ears, nose, throat, the stomach, the bladder, the rectum, etc., much knowledge has been added to what could only be gained by old methods. Electricity especially has been of great use for the purposes of diagnosis and treatment. X-ray analysis, radiology, the electro-cardiogram, ultraviolet rays, ultramicroscopy, infra-red rays, photography, diathermy, etc., have been all very important additions to the plain physical instruments, till now in use. Great advance in diagnostic radiology has been recently made. The radiologist visualises the biliary tract and the gall-bladder by means of certain chemical substances; by injection of air he can outline organs in the abdominal cavity and the sinuses in the brain. By the use of organic compounds of iodine, he can make visible the lungs, the air-passages, the interior of the uterus, etc. Modern fluorescent screen enables digestive movements, heart beats or lung movements to be watched. It cannot yet be said how far physics can be of use to the development of the science of medicine in future. The Āyurvedists must move with the times and make use of the knowledge gained by these instruments for the elucidation of many unexplainable statements found in old literature.

Anumāna **:** अनुमानं नाम तर्को युक्त्यपेक्षः, यथोक्तं, अग्निं जरणशक्त्या, बलं व्यायामशक्त्या, श्रोत्रादीनि शद्बादिग्रहणेनेत्येवमादिः.. ।।-(चरकसंहिता-वि० 8. 6-32)

Anumāna means examination by inference. This involves discrimination between things noticed and association of ideas. All advance in knowledge must consist of both these operations; for, objects first appearing separately, are brought together in the course of our observation. Analysis and synthesis are thus incessantly alternating mental activities without which no ordinary progress in the currency of thought is possible. Reasoning again is an important application of thought to arrive at conclusions, and to know essential and non-essential characters of occurrences. Caraka has made reference to all these mental processes as they are necessary for the proper understanding of the case. The first chapter in *Śarīra-Sthāna* is very important in this respect to study a case and to arrive at a proper diagnosis. For the systematic method of case-taking, this examination is absolutely necessary. Even in the methods of examination by प्रत्यक्ष and आप्तवचन, अनुमान is necessary for discriminating the determinative purposes. For, in *Rasa-Parīkṣā,* we have to depend upon what the patient says regarding the taste in his mouth, or we have to infer the condition of discharges from the way in which insects are attracted to them.

Anumāna again has some scope when one has to judge the condition of the patient from his cravings, mental attitudes, facial expressions, and so on.

Āpta-Vacana तत्राप्तोपदेशोनामाप्तवचनम्, आप्ता ह्यवितर्कस्मृतिविभागविदो निष्प्रीप्युपता-पदर्शिनश्च ।।-(चरकसंहिता-वि० 4.4)

Upadeśa means the rules laid down by experienced clinicians without any restrictions such as formality, faddism or pre-possession. Caraka defines आप्तागम as the advice of disinterested persons whose judgement is well-founded, admitted by scholars and scrutinised by authoritative persons and whose word is only meant for the welfare of humanity परीक्षकै: प्रणीत: शिष्टानुमतो लोकानुग्रहप्रवृत्त: शस्त्रवाद:, स चाऽऽप्तागम: ।। -(चरकसंहिता-सूत्रस्थान 11.27)

It must be noted here that the ancient Āyurvedists who wrote works on medicine, were well-versed in other sciences also such as logic, philosophy, grammar, etc., and so their observations were based on truth and impartial judgement. Though they appreciated the principles laid down in other sciences, they accepted only such of them as would agree with the purposes of medical science. The adjustment of the *Pañcabhautika* theory and formulation of त्रिदोषसिद्धांत show this. They have, similarly, not blindly followed सांख्य, वैशेषिक or न्यायदर्शन but have made such alterations as would suit their purpose. They were aware of the wide range of the way of medical relief, and having kept their mind open to good sense, truth and justice, welcomed all suggestions and deliberations for the sake of human welfare. It was with this object that संभाषापरिषत्s were arranged in olden times. Caraka's words in this connection deserve to be remembered[56] :

So, in other words, *Āpta-vākya* does not only mean blind following but it also means authority proved by facts and tested by experience. In recent times, much is made of such therapeutics which is named 'inductive science' based on observation. Āyurveda does not only accept this, but goes further and makes use of deductive conclusions also, whenever necessary. Therefore, treatment ought to be such that the application of the remedy should be faultless and not one sided. Vāgbhaṭa says,

प्रयोगः शमयेद्व्याधिमेकं योऽन्यमुदीरयेत्।
नाऽसौ विशुद्धः शुद्धस्तु शमयेद्यो न कोपयेत्।।

–(अ.हृ.सू.अ. 13.16)

That medicine which temporarily alleviates symptoms, but may give rise to appearance of disease in some other situation, is not rational, i.e., based on correct principles. But such treatment is appropriate where the medicine modifies but does not, at the same time, provoke new complications.

The theory of tridoṣa

प्रारब्धं यत् स्वयं कार्यं दैवाद् यदि न सिध्यति।
न सीदति च तत् कर्तुमुत्साही च पुनःपुनः।। (2.10.723)

In the Rāja Mānasollāsa more importance is given to उत्साहशक्ति। उत्साहि will not stop, if he experiences loss or fails in his efforts. It says, "The good work begun by the person, if he does not succeed in that work, he must not give up his efforts. He should continue that work with confidence and then he will succeed." According to Rāja Mānasollāsa, a physician must study salient features of *Pancamahābhūtas* and the theory of *Tridoṣa* before the treatment.

Earth, water, fire, air and ether are the five elements or पंचमहाभूतs. The continuation of these five elements is known as प्रकृति or unmanifested nature. प्रकृति evolves from the intellect which is known as महत्, ego—अहंकार—and the five elements are produced by the *Pañcatanmātras.* ज्ञानेन्द्रिय, कर्मेन्द्रिय and मनस् form the five elements. पृथिवी, अप्, अग्नि, वायु and आकाश are the five *Mahābhūtas.*[57] The gross human body or for that matter, the body of any living being, is also composed of five *Mahābhūtas.* The external frame of this universe also has the same material composition. As the source material is the same, there is great similarity between the other universe and the skeleton or the outer frame of any living being.

पंचमहाभूतs or the five elements are supposed to have their own specific qualities. आकाश or ether has no weight. वायु or air is rough. अग्नि or fire is hot. अप् or water is cold. पृथिवी or earth is heavy.[58]

The gross human body is the combination of प्रकृति and पुरुष. पंचमहाभूतs form the प्रकृति which is unmanifest. पुरुष is also the product of the पंचमहाभूतs but he is known to have six components, five Mahābhūtas and the self or जीव. It is the पुरुष who is subjected to medical treatment. A student of medicine is expected to know both प्रकृति and पुरुष minutely for acquainting himself with the structure of human body which forms the study of anatomy and physiology. After carefully examining the structure of the body, one should proceed to find out the cause of disease and disorder and think of preventing or curing the same. After physiology, pathology is the next step in closely observing the cause of disease before undertaking any कायचिकित्सा or medical treatment. It has already been mentioned that it is the पुरुष, the combination of पंचमहाभूतs and the self that is subjected to medical treatment.[59]

शरीर or anatomy and physiology form the foremost basic principle in this science. The meaning of the word शरीर is said to be 'decaying', that which श्रीयते or decays, is known as 'शरीर'. Besides this, देह and काय are also used to denote the physical frame of a living being. काय is also mentioned as the abode of जीव or soul. The body or शरीर is composed of trunk, head and other parts connected with it. त्वक् or the skin covers the whole body. अस्थि bones, support the human body. The human skeleton is bound by several bone joints. पेशि or muscles are attached to bones. नाडीs are attached to the brain and spinal cord. They are spread over the body causing sensation and controlling movements. धमनी—arteries, are channels carrying blood from heart to different organs : सिरा—veins bring the blood back to heart slowly. Between these two are केशिका or capillaries through which रस—nutrient material or serum, oozes to the tissues. हृदय or heart, indicates the three phases receiving, supplying and movement of cardiac cycles. Heart is the main source of life. None can live when it stops. The earliest sages have called it as the seat of consciousness.[60]

Heart is the receptacle of रस and रक्त. It distributes रस and रक्त to the whole body for nourishment and draws out impurities from the same. This is like a lotus situated in the chest. It is flanked by two lungs. Below on the right side is liver and on the left is spleen. Impure blood is purified in the lungs with the help of oxygen drawn in by respiration. Liver is the root of the channels carrying blood and also of पित—bile. पित्त digests the food taken in. Food after digestion is separated as रस—essence and मल the excreta. रस, absorbed from the intestine, goes to heart and मल is expelled from the body.[61] The urine formed in the kidneys is collected in the urinary bladder. शुक्र is seminal vesicle. योनि—female genital tract—is an important seat. Head consists of brain, *prāṇa* and senses and is an important मर्म—sensitive organ. Any injury caused to head, heart, lungs, etc., may prove fatal.

Pañcamahābhūtas—पंचमहाभूतs—no doubt prepare the frame of living bodies; but by themselves they cannot function. After life, enters the body, the three vital principles that are visible in the system, regulate and control its biological functions. वात, पित्त and कफ are the three vital principles which are the subtle forms of the *pañcamahābhūtas*—वायु—(air), अग्नि—(fire), तेजस् and अप्—water, आकाश—ether is too subtle and पृथिवी—earth is too gross. Both of these cannot be involved in any of the above functions.[62] Although every material is composed of the पंचमहाभूतs, there is predominance of any one of them.[63]

वात, पित्त and कफ are considered as त्रिदोषs. Wherever there is life, these three दोषs exist.[64] Every living cell is pervaded by these दोषs. Only then they can function. In all inanimate objects and the dead, there is no function at all. त्रिदोषs are necessarily connected with प्राण or life. These त्रिदोषs cover a wide range of animate groups. It is very interesting to note that वात, पित्त and कफ have each five types of दोषs and each has specific functions of their own as shown below :

	Types of दोष	Function
वात	1. प्राण	Respiration
	2. उदान	Speech
	3. समान	Stimulating digestive fire
	4. व्यान	General movements
	5. अपान	Excretion.[65]
पित्त	1. पाचक	Digestion
	2. रंजक	Pigmentation
	3. भ्राजक	Lustre
	4. आलोचक	Vision
	5. साधक	Energising heart[66]
कफ	1. अवलंबक	Foam in the heart
	2. बोधक	Taste-perception
	3. तर्पक	Saturating Head
	4. क्लेदक	Moistening food
	5. श्लेषक	Uniting joints.[67]

Although all pervasive *doṣas* manifest in certain particular positions, वात manifests below the navel; पित्त between heart and the navel and कफ above the head. According to दृढबलं these three—वात, पित्त and कफ—are influenced by biological and environmental factors and undergo changes. वात, पित्त and कफ increase in old age.[68] Variation of seasons also causes accumulation, aggravation and alleviation. वात, पित्त and कफ are prone to accumulate in summer, aggravate in rainy season and alleviate in autumn respectively.[69] *Doṣas* caused by वात, पित्त and कफ vary according to different seasons. Prevention of these seasonal disorders, requires modification of routine and the physician has to be aware of this fact before starting any treatment.

All the biological functions are controlled by the three *doṣas*. These *doṣas* cannot be restricted to any gross substances as they are all-pervasive. It is for this reason that all biological factors are classified into three groups as वात, पित्त and कफ according to their functions.

An experienced physician knows that the functions of the three *doṣas* depend upon the diet and its nutritive value. Quantity of food is also another important factor to be kept in mind. Along with diet, drugs also have great effect on the three *doṣas*. These drugs are having पंचभौतिकs composition and are mostly influenced by *Rasas* or tastes. The effect of *Rasas* on *doṣas* is indicated by the drugs. *Rasavaisesikasūtra* deals extensively with this point by enumerating the *Rasas* and their characteristics.[70]

Rasas are six in number. मधुर (Sweet), आम्ल (Sour), लवण (Salty), कटु (Pungent), तिक्त (Bitter) and कषाय (Astringent). *Doṣas* are influenced by these. मधुर—(Sweet), is composed of आप् (water) and पृथिवी (earth). It aggravates कफ and pacifies वात and पित्त. आम्ल (Sour) is said to be composed of पृथिवी and अग्नि aggravating पित्त and कफ and pacifying वात. लवण (Salt) is said to be the component of आप् and अग्नि aggravating पित्त and कफ and pacifying वात. पृथिवी is a component in आम्ल and आप् is a component in लवण. The aggravation and pacification in both are the same.[71]

कटु (Pungent), is supposed to be composed of वायु and अग्नि aggravating वात and पित्त and pacifying कफ. तिक्त (Bitter), is having the components of वायु and आकाश aggravating वात and pacifying कफ and पित्त. कषाय (Astringent) is said to be the composition of पृथिवी and वायु aggravating वात and pacifying कफ and पित्त. In तिक्त, आकाश is predominant whereas in कषाय, पृथिवी is prominent. In the same manner, आप् is a component in लवण and वायु is a component in कटु. But in this case, aggravation is पित्त and कफ

whereas, pacification is in वात and लवण. And aggravation in कटु is वात and पित्त and pacification is in कटु.[72]

On closely observing the effect of *Rasas* on *doṣas*, one can make out that each *Rasa* has a positive action, either aggravating or pacifying on two *doṣas*. Each has two predominant पंचमहाभूतs in its composition also. It may be noted that aggravation is another name for वृद्धि or increase and pacification is another name for क्षय or decrease. शीत and उष्ण for that matter are based on अग्नि and सोम of the scriptures. पित्त is increased by उष्ण while शीत increases both कफ and वात.[73]

Āyurveda gives description of धातु (supporting tissues and entities) and मल (excreta) alongside with त्रिदोष. धातु concerned with the digested food in the form of आहाररस (essence of food), is absorbed and carried into the circulation of blood. There is रसधातु in the blood which is nourished by these धातुs. धातुs are mentioned as seven in number such as रस, रक्त, मांस, मेदस्, अस्थि, मज्जा and शुक्र. रस is meant to traverse through arteries which act as irrigating channels through which blood flows. By the essence or आहाररस, धातुs are sustained. मल or excreta is thrown out or discarded by the system in the forms of mucus, dirt, sweat through eyes and skin.[74]

Along with त्रिदोष and धातु, स्रोतस् (arteries or channels) also play an important role in the spread of disorders or disease in the पुरुष. अग्नि is required for transformation or conversion of digested food into आहाररस. Similarly, स्रोतस् is necessary for a continuous flow of आहाररस. Just as any obstruction in the channels dries up a land or field, any hindrance or obstacle in the स्रोतस् causes disorder in the system. Thirteen main channels are described by Caraka and he names them as प्राण (air), उदक (water), अन्न (food); रस, रक्त, मांस मेदस्, अस्थि, मज्जा, शुक्र (which are also referred to as धातुs); मूत्र (urine), पुरीष (faeces) and स्वेद (sweat). Symptoms of their disorder are also stated by him.[75]

Three phases of दोषस्थान–वृद्धि and क्षय and importance of धातु in the System

It is necessary to emphasize here that when प्राण enters the material body, the three *doṣas,* वात, पित्त, कफ, emerge and physiological functions start. वात is composed of air or ether. पित्त consists of heat. कफ is the combination of water with earth.[76] The three *doṣas*—वात, पित्त, कफ—cover the whole system and start functioning from top to bottom of a living body.[77] *Doṣas* define प्रकृति or the human constitution and produce disorders in the living beings.

The three *Doṣas* have characteristics contrary to each other and maintain साम्य or समयोग (equilibrium) in the system. They can be said to behave in the same manner like the three गुणs—सत्व, रजस्, तमस्.[78]

These *doṣas* have a peculiar feature of increase, aggravation or वृद्धि according to age, day and night and intake of food. They must be properly diagnosed and treated. A physician identifies the same according to the qualities of *doṣas* enumerated in the texts. वात has the characteristic of cold, light, subtle and unstable. पित्त is rather hot, sharp, liquid, sour, pungent and moving. कफ is heavy, cold, stable and slimy. When drugs having opposite qualities are administered, these *doṣas* decrease or get pacified and undergo क्षय.[79]

After describing the characteristics, the functions of the three *doṣas* are also enumerated. वात means movement. The normal functions of वात are mentioned as enthusiasm, respiration, transportation of nutrients or धातुs and proper elimination of excreta—

उत्साहो निःश्वासोच्छ्वासौ चेष्टा समा च धातुगतिः।
मलनिर्हरणं सम्यक् वायोः स्यात् प्राकृतं कर्म।।

–(षोडशाङ्गहृदयं-मौ० 43)

The word पित्त is derived from the word ताप which means heat. All functions related to अग्नि are performed by पित्त. Digestion of food, body-heat, thirst and hunger, vision, lustre, cheerfulness and intellect are its natural functions—

आहारपक्तिरूष्मा देहे क्षुत्तृद् तथा समा दृष्टिः।
तेजःप्रसादमेधाः पित्तस्य प्राकृतं कर्म।। *Ibid.*, 45.

श्लेष्मा or कफ has many notable features. श्लिष् is the root from which श्लेष्मा is originated. The meaning of this word is 'to embrace'. Uniting, healing, etc., are, therefore, the functions of कफ. It is supposed to bind by providing firmness, heaviness, virility, strength, etc., to the body. Forbearance, patience and absence of greed are the other functions of कफ–

स्नेहो बन्धः स्थैर्यं गुरुता वृषता बलं ह्यलश्च तनौ।
क्षान्तिर्धृतिस्त्वलोभः कफकर्म प्राकृतं ज्ञेयम्।। *Ibid.*, 47.

The त्रिदोषाः mentioned above along with their qualities and functions have to pass through three phases. They are स्थान or normal status, वृद्धि—increase and क्षय—decrease.[80] Normal functioning of दोषs is said to be the prominent feature of स्थान or natural status. This is an indication of health of a healthy person. Symptoms of disease or disorder are indicated by वृद्धि (increase) or क्षय (decrease). These are considered abnormal states caused by dis-equilibrium or वैषम्य.

Increase, वृद्धि of *doṣas,* is also classified under two categories. One is संचय or accumulation and the other is प्रकोप or aggravation.[81]

The contributory factors for the aggravation of *doṣas* can be listed according to the intake of avoidable diet, variation of age of the human being and the natural seasonal changes.

Intake of rough, bitter and pungent substances in diet causes aggravation. Over eating or undue fasting results in aggravating

वात. Suppression of natural urges and excessive physical exertion increase वात. Intense cold can also be mentioned in this order. Mental worry and keeping awake at night result in excessive वात disorder. In old age, वात normally aggravates. Rainy season is also conducive to वात to shoot up.[82]

Pungent, sour, hot and irritant substances in diet cause पित्त. Anger aggravates पित्त. Young age is prone to be the victim of पित्त disorder. Autumnal season is also mentioned as the reason for increase in पित्त or पित्तविकार. Mid-day and Mid-night are also stated to be the cause of पित्त aggravation.

Excessive intake of sweet, sour, salty, slimy and heavy substances in the diet causes aggravation of कफ. Sleeping in daytime and lack of physical exercise results in the increase of कफ. Childhood is receptive to aggravated कफ. Spring is the season not favourable for कफ to be normal.[83]

It has been mentioned already that *doṣas* get after treatment through drugs having opposite qualities. Qualities of *doṣas* in the mind also should be kept in view before starting any treatment. In order to begin the course of treatment, one should be aware of the symptoms of these *doṣas*. These symptoms of aggravated *doṣas* in वात are found to be pain in abdomen, stiffness, contraction and heaviness in the body, blackish stool, emaciation, loss of sleep; instability, roughness in the skin, irregularity in digestion, abnormal taste, dryness in the mouth etc. After closely observing the symptoms, they have to be eliminated through enema. Then it has to be pacified with the intake of sweet, sour and salty items, rest and sleep. It is said that after treatment, such *doṣas* do not recur.[84]

Pitta is normally caused by heat. As such, burning sensation, unusual perspiration, thirst, yellowishness in skin, eye, urine, etc. are regarded as its symptoms. Purgation is the process of eliminating these symptoms. After treatment, पित्तविकार or प्रकोप

can be pacified by the intake and sprinkling of cold water. Intake of sweet and bitter things, also help in पित्तशमन.

Aggravation of कफ results in heaviness, indigestion, nausea, salivation, drowsiness, excessive sleep, depression of body and mind, etc. Emesis can be used for eliminating the symptoms. Intake of bitter and pungent substances and physical help in pacifying कफ प्रकोप. Application of irritant, hot and rough items also help in this process.

दोषप्रकोप or aggravation of *doṣas* can be made out through abnormal symptoms in the system. Their normal characteristics are absent in the state of क्षय or diminution. In the साम्य or समयोग state *doṣas* conform to their normal functions.[85]

वात, पित्त and कफ are त्रिदोषs necessary for the maintenance of the body. Just as the three *guṇas*—सत्त्व, रजस्, तमस्—with their distinct characteristics maintain equilibrium, the three *doṣas* also with their peculiar characteristic functions, maintain normal status in a healthy body. They also produce abnormality such as वृद्धि—increase and क्षय—decrease. Abnormality is very much pronounced in वृद्धि and weakness in क्षय. Proper identification of the qualities of each दोष is necessary before proceeding on the course of treatment. Each दोष can be treated by a drug having opposite qualities. Symptoms of each *doṣa* are listed so that the physician may easily find out the cause of abnormality and determine the quantum and quality of the drug for eliminating the *doṣa*.

त्रिदोषाs and their different phases form a very important study as they play a vital role in physiology and pathology of living beings. कफ, पित्त and वात may pervade the whole body; but they are particularly located in the head, navel (नाभि:) and below, respectively—

दोषास्त्रयोऽपि देहे व्याप्ताः सकले सदा प्रकुर्वन्ति।
स्वं स्वं कर्म विशिष्टं स्थिताः शिरोनाभ्यधोदेशे।।

(षोडशाङ्गहृदयं.33)

The importance of diet is a prime factor for the drug to act effectively in each case. Over exertion as well as over resting have to be avoided. Normal exercise has to be kept alive so that the diet taken has to be digested and along with the drug gets assimilated in the system of a living being.

Each धातु nourishes the other and in the process undergoes transformation. The last धातु, शुक्र, is produced in a month's period. The essence of all these धातुs is named as ओजस्.[86]

रस is known as 'chyle' in English which means 'a milky fluid formed from chyme by pancreatic juice and bile.'[87] व्यानवायु pumps this रस from हृदय in channels or स्रोतस् to nourish the remaining धातुs. शुक्र which is the last धातु is supposed to take shape in a month's time after undergoing transformation through proper nourishment. शुक्र is not manifested in childhood. It has no capacity to flow in old age.

It is an established fact that Surgical Science is known as a distinct branch of Medicine in Āyurveda.

The practical part of the subject of surgery is preceded by a few general remarks, in which, amidst many erroneous notions, we trace some justness of classification, and soundness of principle. "Living bodies are composed," it is said—

स्वभावमीश्वरं कालं यदृच्छां नियतिं तथा।
परिणामं च मन्यन्ते प्रकृतिः पृथुदर्शिनः।।
तन्मयान्येव भूतानि तद्गुणान्येव चादिशेत्।
तैश्च तल्लक्षणः कृत्स्नो भूतग्रामो व्यजनायत।।

–(सुश्रुतसंहिता–श० 1.11–12)

"Of the five elements, with action or life super added, they are produced from vapour, vegetation, incubation, and parturition, as insects, plants, birds, fishes, reptiles, and animals. Āyurveda considers vegetable bodies as endowed with life. Of animals, man is the chief, and in proportion to his complicated structure is liable to diseae. The disorders of the human frame are of four kinds—accidental, organic, intellectual, and natural. The injuries arising from external causes form the first class. The second comprehends the effects of the vitiated humours, or derangements of the blood, bile, wind, and phlegm. The third class is occasioned by the operation of the passions, or the effects on the constitution of rage, fear, sorrow, joy and others; and the last is referrable to the necessary and innate condition of our being, as thirst, hunger, sleep, old age, and decay.

"The judicious alleviation of human infirmities, the means of which were compassionately revealed by the gods, can only be effected by the knowledge that is to be gained from both study and practice. He who is only well versed in books will be alarmed and confused, like a coward in the field of battle, when he is called upon to encounter active disease. He who rashly engages in practice, without previous conversancy with written science, will be entitled to no respect from mankind, and merits punishment from the king. Those men who, in ignorance of the structure of the human frame, venture to make it the subject of their experiments, are the losers of their species. He alone, who is endowed with both theory and experience, proceeds with safety and stability, like a chariot on two wheels." It is much to be regretted that these aphorisms have so little influence on Āyurveda practitioners.

The instrumental part of medical treatment was, according to the best authorities, of eight kinds—छेदन (*Chhedana*), cutting or scission; भेदन (*Bhedana*), division or excision; लेखन (*Lekhana*), which means drawing lines. व्याधन (*Vyādhana*), puncturing; एश्या (*Eśya*), probing, or sounding; अहार्य (*Ahārya*), extraction of solid bodies, विस्रावण (*Visrāvaṇa*), extraction of fluids, including venesection; and सेवन (*Sevana*), or sewing; and the mechanical means, by which these operations were performed, seem to have been sufficiently numerous. Of these, the principal are the following :

यन्त्रा (*Yantras*), properly machines, in the present case instruments; but to distinguish them from the next class, to which that title more particularly applies, we may call them implements; शस्त्रा (*Śastrās*), weapons, or instruments; क्षार (*Kṣāra*), alkaline solutions, or caustics; अग्नि (*Agni*), fire, the actual cautery; शलाका (*Śalākā*), pins, or tents; श्रृङ्ग (*Śringa*), horns, the horns of animals open at the extremities, and as well as अलाबू (*Alābū*), or gourds, used as our cupping glasses; the removal of the atmospheric pressure through the first being effected by suction, and in the second by rarifying the air by the application of a lamp. The next subsidiary means are जलौका *(Jalaukā)*, or leeches.

Besides these, we have thread, leaves, bandages, pledgets, heated metallic plates for erubescents, and a variety of astringent or emollient applications. The enumeration is tolerably full, and the details are curious, if not instructive.

A few instruments, and some of neat and ingenious fabric, are in the hands of native operators, particularly those for depressing cataracts; but they are not very common.

We can only therefore conjecture what the instruments might have been, by adding to the imperfect description given of them the purport of their names, and the objects to which they were applied.

The *Yantras,* or implements, known to Suśruta (I, Ch. 7) were one hundred and one, and were classed as *Swastikas, Sandanśas, Tālayantras, Nāḍiyantras, Śalākās* and *Upayantras.*

तत्र, मनः शरीराबाधकराणि शल्यानि; तेषामाहरणोपायो यन्त्राणि।।

तानि षट्प्रकाराणिः, तद्यथा-स्वस्तिकयन्त्राणि, संदंशयन्त्राणि, तालयन्त्राणि, नाडियन्त्राणि, शलाकायन्त्राणि, उपयन्त्राणि, चेति।।

तत्र चतुर्विंशतिः स्वस्तिकयन्त्राणि, द्वे संदंशयन्त्रे, द्वे एव तालयन्त्रे विंशतिर्नाड्यः अष्टाविंशतिः शलाकाः, पञ्चविंशतिरुपयन्त्राणि।। तानि प्रायशो लौहानि भवन्ति, तत्प्रतिरूपकाणि वातदलाभे। तत्र, नानाप्रकारा भवन्ति,

तत्प्रतिरूपकाणि वातदलाभे। तत्र, नानाप्रकाराणां व्यालानां मृगपक्षिणां मुखैर्मुखानि यन्त्राणां...।।

(सुश्रुतसंहिता-सूत्रस्थानम् 7.4-10)

The *Swastikas* are twenty four in number—they are metallic, usually eighteen inches long, having heads or points fancifully shaped like the heads of animals, the beaks of birds, etc. They are secured with small pins, and are curved or hooked at the points, and are used to extract splinters of bone or foreign bodies lodged in the bones—they were, therefore, pincers, nippers, or forceps.

The *Sandansās,* which in usual import mean tongs, were of that description. There were in the time of Suśruta but two sorts, one with and the other without a ligature or noose (*Nigraha*?) attached. They were smaller than the preceding, being sixteen inches in length; and were used to remove extraneous substances from the soft parts, as the flesh, skin, vessels. The work of Vāgbhaṭa adds another sort, only six inches long, which were employed preferably for the soft parts and for fleshy excrescences.

The *Tālayantras* must have been something of the same kind, only smaller, their length being but twelve inches. They were but two, and were employed to remove foreign matters lodged in the outer canals, as the ears.

The *Nāḍiyantras* were, as the name implies, tubular instruments. There were twenty sorts, varying in size and shape according to their intended use. They were employed for removing extraneous bodies from deep seated canals, as the intestines, urethra. For examining affections of parts similarly removed from inspection; for the introduction of other instruments, so as to enable them to be applied; and for drawing off fluids by suction. The work of Vāgbhaṭa specifies the number of perforations in each of these tubes, as they varied in this respect as well as others : the descriptions are, however, very indistinct, and we can only conclude generally, that they bore an analogy to our catheters, syringes, etc.

The *Śalākās* were hollow round rods. They were of twenty-eight kinds, varying in size and shape, for extracting foreign matters, lodged in parts of difficult access; for cleansing or clearing internal canals, especially the urethra; for applying collyria, caustic solutions, and the actual cautery; and for eradicating nasal polypi, the complaint called *Nakra* so common and so troublesome in India, and to be alleviated by no other means than the forcible extraction of the irritating excrescence.

The *Upayantras* were, as their appellation signifies, merely accessory implements, such as twine, leather, bark, skin, cloth. The first, best, and most important of all implements, however, is declared to be the hand. *Śastras,* the instruments, of which twenty different sorts are enumerated as under :

विंशतिः शस्त्राणि, तद्यथा-मण्डलाग्र करपत्र वृद्धिप्रपत्र नखशस्त्रमुद्रिकोत्पलपत्र।

यदा सुनिशितं शस्त्रं रोमच्छेदि सुसंस्थितम्।

सुगृहीतं प्रमाणेन तदा कर्मसु योजयेत्।। (सुश्रुतसंहिता-सूत्रस्थानं 8.3-14)

They were of metal, and always bright, handsome, polished, and sharp; sufficiently so indeed to divide a hair longitudinally. Vāgbhaṭa however, adds, they were in general not above six inches in length, and that the blade formed about a half or quarter of that length.

Thus, the different kinds of scission, longitudinal, transverse, inverted, and circular, are directed to be practised on flowers, bulbs, and gourds. Incision on skins, or bladders, filled with paste and mire;—scarification on the fresh hides of animals from which the hair has not been removed;—puncturing, or lancing, on the hollow stalks of plants, or the vessels of dead animals;—extraction on the cavities of the same, or fruits with many large seeds, as the Jack and Bel;—sutures, on skin and leather, and ligatures and bandages on well-made models of the human limbs.

The employment of leather, skin, and even of dead carcases, thus enjoined, proves an exemption from notions of impurity. Of course, their use implies the absence of any objections to the similar employment of human subjects. Although they are not specified, they may possibly be implied, in the general direction which Suśruta gives, that the teacher shall seek to perfect his pupil by the application of all expedients which he may think calculated to effect his proficiency.

References

1. M.N. Joshi, *Principles of* Āyurveda, *chapter* 'आदर्श राष्ट्रस्य वैदिकी कल्पना', Roopa Publications, Dharwad, 1999, pp. 222-23.
2. M.N. Joshi, *op.cit.*, p. 27.
3. *Ibid.*,
4. *Ibid.*, pp. 32-33.
5. *Ibid.*, p. 34.
6. *Ibid.*, p. 37.
7. Henry E. Sigerist, *A History of Medicine* Vol. II, (Oxford University Press, New York, 1961), p. 137.
8. *Ibid.*, p. 143.
9. *Ibid.*, p. 144.
10. We see in particular the healing feats of the twin horsemen, Aśvins at Ṛg-Veda 1.112.8, 15· 116.10, 15, 16; 117.9, 13, 17-18, 24; 118.6-8; 5.74.5; 75.5; 7.68.6; 71.5; 10.39.3, 4, 8; and 10.40.5; the connection of Rudra with healing at Ṛg-Veda 1.43.4; 114.5; 2.33.2, 4, 7, 12; 5.42.11; 7.35.6; 46.3; and 8.29.5; of the Maruts at Ṛg-Veda 2.33.13; and 8.20.23-26; of Soma and Rudra at Ṛg-Veda 6. 74.3; of Indra at Ṛg-Veda 2.21.6; 4.19.9; 8.1.12 and especially 8.91(80), where Indra cures Apāla of the loss of hair and of ugly skin.
11. A.F. Rudolf Hoernle, *Studies in the Medicine of Ancient India,* Part I : Osteology or the Bones of the Body (Oxford : Clarendon Press, 1907); Frederick S. Hammett, "The Anatomical Knowledge of the Ancient Hindus," *Annals of Medical History* (New Series) 1 (1929) : 325-33; and Jean Filliozat, La doctrine pp. 117-37.
12. M.N. Joshi, *op.cit.* pp. 58-59, Roopa Publications, Dharwad, 1999.
13. *Ibid.*, pp. 60-61.
14. *Ibid.*, p. 6.
15. *Ibid.*, pp. 73-74.

16. शिवशेखरमिश्र, मानसोल्लास-एक सांस्कृतिक अध्ययन (Chowkhamba Vidyabhavan, Varanasi, 1996, पृ० 196-203.
17. हिरण्यं च मे श्श्चमे सीसं चमे त्रपुश्चमे श्यामं च मे लोहं च मे। (यजुर्वेद 14.13)
18. D.D. Mehta, *Positive Science in the Vedas*, Arnold Heinemann, New Delhi, 1974, p. 47.
19. गीतम् वाद्यम् नृत्यम् आलोख्यम् विशेषकच्छेद्यम्....
    ....रूप्यरत्नपरीक्षा धातुवादः...।। (वात्स्यायन कामसूत्र 1.3.16)
20. वेगानां धारणादोजः स्नेहशुक्रक्षयादपि।
    अपिव्यायामतो हीनः श्वास कास ज्वरामयः।। (1.19.212)
    क्षाराम्ललवणैर्द्रव्यैरविद्युक्तैः श्रमादपि।
    आतपाच्च भृशं पित्तं कुपितं दूषयेदतृक्।। (1.19.200)
    विरुद्धेनान्नपानेन साधूनां निन्दया वधात्।
    प्राक्तनैः कर्मभिः क्रूरैः कुष्टं श्वित्रं च जायते।। (2.19.272)
    Cf. चरकसंहिता सूत्रस्थाान, 7. 3-5
    न वेगान् धारयेद्धीमाञ्जातान् मूत्रपुरीषयोः।
    न रेतसो न वातस्य न छर्क्षाः क्षयर्थोर्न च।।
    नोद्गारस्य न जृम्भाया न वेगान् क्षुत्पिपासयोः।
    न वाष्पस्य न निद्राया निःश्वासस्य श्रमेण च।।
    एतान् धारयतो जातान् वेगान् रोगा भवन्ति ये।
    पृथक्पृथक्चिकित्सार्थं तान्मे निगदतः श्रुणु।।
21. सामो दोषश्चिराद् हत्वा पावकं जठरस्थितम्।
    निरुध्य च ससञ्चारमुदराग्निं बहिः क्षिपेत्।।
    एवं विनिर्गतो बहिः कायमाश्रित्य तापयन्।
    ज्वर इत्युच्यते तज्वैः सर्वव्याधिपतिश्च सः।। (1.19.145-146)
22. संख्यातावद्यथा अष्टौ ज्वराः, पञ्चगुल्माः, तप्रा कुष्ठाप्येवमादिः।
    (चरकसंहिता-निदानस्थान 1.2)
23. बिल्वं बला पृथक्पर्णीं नागरं धान्यकोत्पलम्।
    एतैः पेया कृता देया वातपित्तज्वरापहा।। (1.19.160)
24. मूर्वा-निम्ब-पटोलातिविष-धन्वयवासकैः।
    शुण्ठी-मुस्तामृतायासैः क्वाथौ वातज्वरापहः।। (1.19.185)
25. अथ क्षल्वष्टाभ्योः कारणेभ्यो ज्वरः संजायते मनुष्याणां, तद्यथा-वातात्, पित्तात्, कफात्, वातपित्ताभ्यां, वातकफाभ्यां, पित्तकफाभ्यां, वातपित्तकफेभ्यः, आगन्तोरष्टमात् कारणात्।।
    (चरकसंहिता-निदानस्थान 1.17)
26. ज्वरो नरेषु विख्यातः पालकः सामजन्मसु।
    अभितापस्तुरङ्गेषु वारको रासभेष्वसौ।।
    उष्ट्रेष्वलसकः प्रोक्तो गोषु प्रोक्तस्तथेश्वरः।
    अक्षिको दन्दशूकेशु हारिद्रो महिषेष्वपि।।

अजाविको प्रलेपस्स्यान्मृगरोगो मृगेष्वपि।
अवपातः शकुन्तेषु मत्स्येष्विन्द्रमदाभिधः।।
गुल्मेषु ग्रन्थिको ज्योतिर्वनस्पत्यौषधीष्वपि।।
पुष्पेषु पर्वतः प्रोक्तो रूपको नलिनीष्वपि।।
धान्येषु चूर्णकः ख्यातः कोद्रवेषु ललः स्मृतः।
शाकेषु मधुको भूम्यामूषरोऽप्यु च नीलिका।। (2.6.639-643)

27. एकभक्तं तथा पेया मण्डो वा कोष्णवारिणा।
दोषकोपानुसारेण लङ्घनं विविधं स्मृतम्।। (1.19.153)

28. सक्तुपिष्टकमश्नीयात् पिबेश्च स्वादु पानकम्।
घृतं वा केवलं पीतं मदात्ययहरं परम्।। (1.19.225)
Cf. महाभारत शान्तिपर्व 309.18
विरक्तस्य यथा सम्यग् घृतं भवति भेषजम्।
तथा निर्हृतदोषस्य प्रेत्य धर्मः सुखावहः।।

29. यथा प्रज्वलितं वेश्म परिषिञ्चन्ति वारिणा।
नराः शान्तिमभिप्रेत्य तथा जीर्णज्वरे घृतम्।। (चरकसंहिता निदानस्थान 1.38)

30. ततो घ्राणस्य कर्णेभ्यः पायु-मेहनमार्गतः।
प्रवर्तते ततः ख्यातं रक्तपित्तं भिषग्वरैः।।
एकदोषं नवं चोर्ध्वं बलिनश्चानुपद्रवम्।
रक्तपित्तं सुखात् साध्यमधश्चेद् याप्यमुच्यते।।
अधश्चोर्ध्वं च चलितं त्रिदोषं भूर्युपद्रवम्।
असाध्यं रक्तपित्तं तत् त्यजनीयं भिषग्वरैः।। (1.19.201-203)

31. तत्रासाध्यं परित्याज्यं याप्यं यत्नेन यापयेत्।
साध्यं चावहितः सिद्धैर्भेषजैः साधयेद्भिषक्।। (चरकसंहिता निदानस्थान 2.27)

32. श्यामा त्रिवृत्कषायेण तत्कल्केन सितान्वितम्।
लोहं विपाचितं दद्यात् कर्शमात्रमसृग्हरम्।।
पिप्पली त्रिफला श्यामा शर्करा त्रिवृता मधु।
एतैः कृतो मोदकोऽयं सन्निपातोत्थरक्तजित्।। (1.19.204-205)

33. भृशं प्रकुपितो वातः कफपित्तमुदीरयेत्।
देहसन्धीन् समाविश्य क्षयरोगं समावहेत्।।
रास्ना-तिल-बलाचूर्णं ससर्षिर्यष्टिकोत्पलम्।
अवलीढं हरेच्छेषमग्निमान्द्यं च नाशयेत्।। (1.19.213-214)

34. अनिष्टान्नोपयोगेन मारुतः कुपितो भृशम्।
उदानं कुरुते छर्दं नाभिपृष्ठरुजान्विताम्।। (1.19.215)

35. जम्बू-चूत-बलोशीर-वटशुङ्गावरोहजः।
क्षौद्रेण सहितः क्वाथः पीतश्छर्दिविनाशनः।। (1.19.217)

36. हीनमिथ्यातिपानेन भवत्याषु मदात्ययः।
छर्दिर्मोहो भ्रमस्तन्द्रा प्रलापो जायते ततः।। (1.19.218)

37. पञ्चाहं सप्तरात्रं वा जायतेऽसो मदात्यय:।
अत ऊर्ध्वं प्रसक्तश्चेद् रोगोऽन्य: परिकीर्त्यते।। (1.19.219)
38. स्वाप: प्रलापबहुले योजनीयो मदात्यये।
छाग-तित्तिर-लावैण-शशमांसरसैर्युतम्।।
सक्तुपिष्टकमश्नीयात् पिबेच्च स्वादु पानकम्।
घृतं वा केवलं पीतं मदात्ययहरं परम्।। (1.19.224-225)
39. गुदान्त्रवलिसम्भूता विष्टाधारणहेतुका:।
अङ्कुरा: कथिता: प्राज्ञैरर्शसीत्यभिधानत:।। (1.19.226)
40. शृङ्गी हरीतकी-कुष्ट-भल्लातकफलै: कृतै:।
लेपस्तुत्थसमोपेतो गुदकीलविनाशन:।। (1.19.227)
41. मूलै: शिग्रुभवैर्बीजैर्निम्बाश्वत्थदलैरपि।
बिल्वेन पीलुमूलेन रामठेनापि लेपनम्।। (1.19.228)
42. सिंहले तु भवेद् रक्तं पद्मरागमनुत्तमम्।
पीतं कालपुरोद्भूतं कुरुविन्दमिति स्मृतम्।।
अशोकपल्लवच्छायमान्ये सौगन्धिकं विदु:। (2.4.475-476)
43. क्षीरमध्ये क्षिपेन्नीलं दुग्धं चेन्नीलतां व्रजेत्।
इन्द्रनील: स विज्ञेयो रविनन्दनवल्लभ:।। (2.4.505)
44. गौरवं स्वच्छता कान्ति: काठिन्यं रत्नजा गुणा:।। (2.4.531)
45. दोषैस्त्यक्तो गुणैर्युक्त इन्द्रनीलो महामणि:।
यस्य हस्ते भवेत् तस्य वित्तमायुर्बलं यश:।। (2.4.504)
46. सेवालवल्लरीच्छायं सुरङ्गं त्रासवर्जितम्।
अनर्घ्यं तं मरकतं प्राहु: सर्व विषापहरम्।। (2.4.518)
47. अत्यम्बुपानाज्जायेत सुतरामतिसाररुक्। आम: पक्व: सरकश्च त्रिधाऽसौ व्याधिरीरित:।।
तत्रामे नागरं मुस्ता तथा च घुणवल्लभा। तच्चूर्णं वटक: दवाथ: पाचनाय प्रयुज्यते।।
(1.19.230-231)
48. पक्वातिसारे दातव्यं जम्बूपल्लव-धातकी। जीरकं चूतबीजं च महावृक्षत्वचस्तथा।।
बिल्वारनाल-गोकण्ट-पञ्चाङ्गुलयवै: शृता। स्विन्ना पथ्या पक्वतीसारभैषजम्।।
(1.19.232-233)
49. विषा कुटजबीजं च मुस्ता वालक-बिल्वकम्।
तत्क्वाथो विनिहन्त्याशु रक्तातीसारमुल्बणम्।। (1.19.234)
50. उरुबूको बला बिल्वं पञ्चमूलद्वयं यवा।
पुनर्नवा भीरुमूलं कुलत्थं बदरं तथा।।
मत्स्याक्षं-मत्स्यभेदं च तत् सर्वं च समं कृतम्।
सत्क्वाथेन सकल्केन सर्पिस्तैलयुतेन च।।
सूकरस्याच्छभल्लस्य वसया मिश्रितेन च।
पञ्चभिर्लवणै: सार्द्धं शूलं पीतेन हन्यते।। (1.19.240-242)

51. आगन्तुर्हि व्यथापूर्वं समुत्पन्नो जघन्यं वातपित्तश्लेष्मणां वैषम्यमापादयति, निजे तु वातपित्तश्लेष्माण: पूर्वं वैषम्यमापद्यन्ते जघन्य व्यथामभिनिर्वर्तयान्ति।। (चरकसंहिता- सूत्रस्थान 20.7)

52. यदातु रक्तवाहीनि रससंज्ञावहानि च।
पृथक्पृथक्समस्ता वा स्रोतांसि कुपिता मला:।।
मलिनाहारशौलस्य रजोमोहावृतात्मन:।
प्रतिहत्यावतिष्ठन्ते जायन्ते व्याधयस्तदा।। (चरकसंहिता-सूत्रस्थान 24.25-26)

53. चय एव जयेद्दोषं कुपितं त्वविरोधयन्।
सर्वकोपे बलीयांसं शेषदोषाविरोधत:।। (अष्टाङ्ग हृदयम् सू.अ. 13.15)

54. समदोष: समाग्निश्च समधातुमलक्रिय:।
प्रसन्नात्मेंद्रियमना: स्वस्थ इत्यभिधीयते।। (सुश्रुतसंहिता-सूत्रस्थान 15.48)

55. एतादेव हिभैषज्यप्रयोगे फलमिष्टं स्वस्थवृत्तानुष्ठाने च यावद्धातूनां साम्यं स्यात्।। (चरकसंहिता-शा० 6.7)

56. न चैव ह्यस्ति सुतरामायुर्वेदस्य पारम्, तस्मादप्रमत्त: शश्वदभियोगमस्मिन् गच्छेत्, एतद्धा कार्यमेवंभूयश्च वृत्तसौष्टवमनसूयता परेभ्योऽप्यागमयितव्यम्।। (चरकसंहिता-वि० 8.6)

57. प्रकृतिप्रवर्तितेयं संसृतिरखिला, ततो महान् जात:।
महतश्चाहंकारोऽहङ्कारात् पञ्चतन्मात्रम्।।
एकादशेन्द्रियाणि श्रवणाद्यर्थानि चाथ जायन्ते।
तन्मात्रेभ्यो भूतानि वियद्वाय्वम्बुसलिलधरा:।। (1.2.5-26)
-षोडशाङ्गहृदयम्-P.V. Sharma.

58. खं वायुरग्निराप: पृथिवी चैतानि पञ्चभूतानि।
लघुतारौक्ष्यञ्चौष्ण्यं शैत्यं गुरुता गुणास्तेषाम्।। (तदेव 27)

59. षड्धात्वात्मकसंज्ञ: पञ्चमहाभूतजीवसमवाय:।
पुरुषो वैद्यकशास्त्रे मतश्चिकित्साक्रियाधिकृत:।। (तदेव 28)

60. षोडशाङ्गहृदयम्-'शारीरम्' P.V. Sharma pp. 180-181.

61. षोडशाङ्गहृदयम्-'शारीरम्' P.V. Sharma, Chapter II pp. 14-15.

62. तत्रास्य केचिदङ्गावयवा मातृजादीनवयवान् विभज्य पूर्वमुक्ता यथावत्। (चरकसंहिता- शरीरस्थान 4-12)

63. सूक्ष्मरूक्षखरशिशिरलघुविशदं स्पर्शबहुलमीषत्तिक्तं विशेषत:...। (सुश्रुतसंहिता-सूत्रस्थान 41.3)

64. नित्या: प्राणभृतां देहे वातपित्तकफास्त्रय:।
विकृता: प्रकृतिस्था वातान् बुभुत्सेत पण्डित:।। (चरकसंहिता-सूत्रस्थान 18-48)

65. तेषां तु मलप्रसादाख्यानां धातूनां स्त्रोतांस्ययनमुखानी। तानि... (चरकसंहिता-सूत्रस्थान 28, 5-11)

66. तच्चादृष्टहेतुकेन विशेषेण पक्वामाशयमध्यस्थं पित्तं....... (सुश्रुतसंहिता-सूत्रस्थान 21-10)

67. श्लोष्मा तु पञ्चधा उर: स्थ: स त्रिकस्य स्ववीर्यत।... (अष्टंगहृदयं-सूत्रस्थान 12-15-18)

68. वयोऽहोरा त्रिभुक्तानां तेऽन्तमध्यादिगा: क्रमात्।

68. वयोऽहोरा त्रिभुक्तानां तेऽन्तमध्यादिगा: क्रमात्।
तैर्भवेद्विषमस्तीक्ष्णो मन्दश्चाग्नि: समै: सम:।। (अष्टांगहृदयं-सूत्रस्थान 1-8)
69. चयप्रकोपशमा: पित्तादीनां यथाक्रमम्।
भवन्त्येकैकश: षट्सु कालेष्वभ्रागमादिषु।। (चरकसंहिता-सूत्रस्थान 17-114)
70. रसनार्थो रससास्य द्रव्यमाप: क्षितिस्तथा।
निर्वतौ च विशेषे च प्रत्यमा: स्वादयस्त्रय:।। (चरकसंहिता-सूत्रस्थान 1.64)
71. वृद्धि: समानै: सर्वेषां विपरीतैर्विपर्यय:।
रसा: स्वाद्वम्ललवणतिक्तोषणकषायक:।।
षड् द्रव्यमाश्रितास्ते च यथापूर्वं बलावह:।
तत्राद्या मारुतं घ्नन्ति त्रस्तिक्तादय: कफम्।। (अङ्गांगहृदय-सूत्रस्थान 1.14-15)
72. *Ibid.*, 10.1, 6-21.
73. नेत्याहुरन्ये, वीर्य प्रधानमिति।... (सुश्रुतसंहिता-सूत्रस्थान 40-5)
74. तत्राहारप्रसादाख्यो रस: किट्टं च मलाख्यमभिर्निवर्तते।
(चरकसंहिता 'सूत्रस्थान' 28.4; चिकित्सास्थान 15.18-19).
75. विसर्गे पुनर्वायवो नातिरूक्षा: प्रवान्ति, इतरे पुनरादाने, सोमश्चाव्याहतबल: शिशिराभिर्भाभिरा-
पुरयजगदाप्याययति शश्वत्, अतो विसर्ग: सौम्य:।। *Ibid.*, 6.5-9.
76. प्राणानां संयोगात् वपुषि जडे पञ्चभूतनिष्पन्ने।
जीवनवृत्तिस्थित्यौ सञ्जायन्ते त्रयो दोष:।।
वायुनभोभ्यां वात:, पित्तं त्वग्रेस्तथा भवेच्छलेष्मा।
अप्पृथिवीभ्यां द्वाभ्यामित्थं तेषां समुत्पत्ति:।।
-षोडशाङ्गहृदयम्-मौलिकसिद्धाता:—P.V. Sharma, 30-31.
77. दोषास्त्रयोऽपि देहे व्याप्ता: सकले सदा प्रकुर्वन्ति।
स्वं स्वं कर्म विशिष्टं स्थिता: शिरोनाभ्यधोदेश:। *Ibid.*, 33.
78. त्रिगुणा इव त्रिदोषा अन्योन्यविपर्यस्वरूपभृत:।
साम्यस्थापनकुशला: चित्र कृतस्ते हि शैलूषा:।। *Ibid.*, 36.
79. रूक्ष: शीतो लघुरथ सूक्ष्मोऽत्यन्तं चलस्तथा विशद:।
खरतावां श्रापि गुणैर्वायुर्विज्ञैर्विनिर्दिष्ट:।।
ईषत्स्निग्धञ्चोष्णं तीक्ष्णं द्रवमम्लभावसंयुक्तम्।
सरमय कटुत्वासहितं पित्तं तज्ज्ञै: गुणै: प्रोक्तम्।।
गौरवशैत्यसुमार्दवसुस्वादुत्वै सुहृत्सम: स्निग्ध:।
स्थिरपिच्छिलञ्च गुणत: श्लेष्मा प्रोक्तो भिषग्वर्यै:।।
विपरीतैस्तुगुणेभ्यो भेषजकल्पै: प्रशान्तिमुपयान्ति।
इति दोषगुणान् धृत्वा मनसि भिषक् कर्म कुर्वीत।।
-षोडशाङ्गहृदयम्-मौलिकसिद्धाता:—P.V. Sharma, 38-41.
80. 'दोषगति: स्यात् त्रिविधा स्थानं, वृद्धि क्षयस्तृतीयञ्च।
'षोडशाङ्गहृदयम्-मौलिकसिद्धान्ता:'।। 48
81. वृद्धिश्चापि द्विविधा सञ्चयरूप: प्रकोपश्च। *Ibid.*, 48.

82. रुक्षेस्तिक्तकषायैः कटुभिरनशनैश्च वेगसंरोधैः।
व्यायामात्त्वतिशैत्यात् धातुःह्रासान् मनः सादात्।।
रात्रौ जागरणादपि प्रवृट्काले तथा च वार्धक्ये।
राव्याश्चरसे सायं चान्ने जीर्णेऽनिलक्षो।। *Ibid.*, 52-53.

83. मधुराम्ललवणसहितैर्द्रव्यैः सुस्निग्धपिच्छलैर्गुरुभिः।
स्वापाद् दिवसे काले स्वभावतः पुष्पसमये च।।
दिवसस्याद्यो भागे रात्र्याश्चापि श्रमातिराहित्यात्।
बाल्ये वयसि प्रकोपो भवति कफस्यापि धीरस्य।। *Ibid.*, 56-57.

84. कोपे वातस्य भवेच्छूलं जठरे रुजा तथाऽङ्गेषु।
स्तब्धत्वं संकोचः कर्कशता कृष्णताविट्सु।। *Ibid.*, 58.

85. मधुराम्ललवणयोगैर्वातं स्नेहेन मित्रवच्छमयेत्।
बहुशः स्वेदविधानात् विश्रामान्तिद्रया हर्षैः।।
मधुरैर्तिक्तकषायैः पित्तं स्थानं निजंद्रुतं व्रजति।
सान्त्वनया सुहृदामपि शीतलजलपानसेकाभ्याम्।।
द्रव्यैः तिक्तकषायैः कटुभिःश्लेष्मा शमं समायाति।
तीक्ष्णोष्णरुक्षयोगैः जागरणाच्चेष्टया चापि।।
कुपिता जनयन्ति रुजः क्षीणाः दोषाः स्वलक्षणं जहति।
साम्यावस्थाप्राप्ताः प्रकृताः स्वं कुर्वते कर्म।। *Ibid.*, 66-69.

86. रसरक्तमांसमेदोऽस्थितदन्तर्भूतमज्जशुक्राणि।
धारणपोषणकरणात् सप्तै ते धातवः ख्याताः।।
रसप्रभृतीनां तेषां धातूनां सार ओज इति विदितः।
तद्व्याधिप्रतिबन्धकबलरूपं श्लेष्मलिङ्गच्च।।
रसधातुहृदयस्थो व्यानक्षिप्तः शरीरधमनीषु।
कुल्यास्विव केदारीं धातूनङ्गानि पोषयति।।
धात्वाहाराः काले परिणामं धातवः सदा यान्ति।
एवं चरमो धातुः शुक्रं मासेन संभवति।।
–षोडशाङ्गहृदयम्–मौलिकसिद्धांता:–70-73, P.V. Sharma p. 176.

87. *Concise Oxford Dictionary*, New Edition, p. 140.

3

BASIC CONCEPTS OF ĀYURVEDA

Āyurveda is the Veda of Āyuṣ, 'आयुष्'. This science of life has come down from the earliest times in India. The great scholar-physician Caraka says that it was revealed by Brahman, the Creator Himself.[1] According to Suśruta, Āyurveda was revealed even before creation.[2] Scholars are of the opinion that Āyurveda is an *Upaveda* related either to Ṛgveda or Atharvaveda. Kaśyapa considers it as the fifth Veda occupying the topmost position.[3] Caraka is emphatic on the point that Āyurveda is शाश्वत—eternal—and its origin is not easy to trace.

A distinctive part of Vedic medicine is its pharmacopoeia, especially its detailed description of the substances and its acquaintance with the local flora. This botanical wisdom occurs largely in the hymns of the Atharvaveda and is connected to a tradition of healing plant goddesses. The hymns of the Ṛgveda reveal less of a familiarity with indigenous plant life, and what is found there relates principally to a tradition of a male plant divinity. A homologization of these two botanical traditions is reflected in the mythological connections between the principal plant deities mentioned in each text, and occurs in mythical parts of the Atharvavedic medical hymns. Here are found myths of both the healing plant god Kuṣṭha, and the healing plant goddess Arundhatī. Kuṣṭha was the remedy *par excellence* for fever. This was generally identified with the aromatic costus, native of Kashmīr and known to have been an important export from India in the spice trade. The healing plant goddess Arundhatī was used in the treatment of fractures and wounds and is identified among others with *lākṣā,* the Sanskrit term for the resinous "lac." The mythology of Kuṣṭha plant god links him closely both with the Ṛgvedic plant Soma, important to the sacrificial cults, and the Atharvavedic Arundhatī, significant to the medical cults. He (Kuṣṭha) is called Soma's brother, and like Soma, is known to have grown high in the Himavant mountains, the birthplace of eagles, the third heaven from earth and the seat of the gods. Likewise, several of the epithets associated with Kuṣṭha are identical to those given to Arundhatī. They are both perennial, life-giving and harmless. Kuṣṭha's mythological link with Soma and his name-association with Arundhatī imply a conscious effort to homologize a Ṛgvedic botanical tradition dominated by a male plant divinity with a medical-botanical tradition of plant goddesses particular to the Atharvaveda.[4] This assimilation of useful (and thereby powerful) botanical knowledge concurs with the medical intellectuals' general tendency to appropriate wisdom which could render their healing rituals more efficacious. Further investigations of the mythological traditions of plant divinities in the Ṛgveda and Atharvaveda should reveal interesting aspects of the homologization of religious ideas and help identify elements of indigenous beliefs in ancient India.

Āyurvedaśāstra : It is definitely known that sciences in India had developed and achieved great eminence at a time when Europe was passing through the dark period of the early middle ages. It is through the medium of the Arabian sciences that some of those Indian scientific concepts and inventions joined the mainstream of the Renaissance in Europe. A few notable names associated with different sciences in India during different periods are given below.[5]

S.No.	*Scientist*	*Period and Profession*
1.	Bharadvāja	Around 800 B.C. Earliest teacher of Āyurvedic Medicine.
2.	Ātreya	8th Century B.C. Renowned teacher of Āyurvedic medicine.
3.	Śālihotra	8th Century B.C. Father of Ancient Indian Veterinary Sciences.
4.	Jīvika	6th Century B.C. Physician to Lord Buddha.
5.	Patañjali	2nd Century B.C. Expounder of the Yoga doctrine.
6.	Caraka	2nd Century B.C. Physician who compiled a treatise on Āyurvedic medicine, known as *Carakasaṁhitā.*
7.	Suśruta	1st Century B.C. Surgeon, who compiled a treatise known as *Suśruta-saṁhitā.*
8.	Vāgbhaṭa	6th Century A.D. A great Physician and Author of *Aṣṭāṅga Hṛdaya* a classic of Āyurvedic Medicine.
9.	Mādhavaka	9th Century A.D. Clinical diagnostician.
10.	Vṛnda	10th Century A.D. Āyurvedic Medicine, practitioner.
11.	Gadāvara Miśra	12th Century A.D. Veterinary Scientist.
12.	Lagadha	9th Century B.C. The first known Astronomer.
13.	Baudhāyana	5th Century B.C. The Geometer (land measurer) of the Vedic Atlas.
14.	Garga	3rd Century B.C. The enumerator of the constellations.

15.	Āryabhaṭṭa	476 A.D. The great Mathematician.
16.	Varāhamihīra	499 A.D. Versatile Scientist. The great Astrologer.
17.	Brahmagupta	598 A.D. A great Mathematician.
18.	Bhāskara	1114 A.D., Algebraist.
19.	Nāgārjuna	8th Century A.D. Great Alchemist.
20.	Kaṇāda	6th Century B.C. Ancient Atomist philosopher/scientist.
21.	Kapila	7th Century B.C. Propounder of the theory of the creation of the universe.
22.	Gotama	6th Century B.C. Originator of Ancient Indian Scientific Methodology.
23.	Khana	6th century B.C. Agriculture.

On the basis of the above information, it may be surmised that science was divided into many parts and intensively studied.

The wrod *Śāstra* was originally applied to the various subjects of study connected with the Vedic religion and Hindu Philosophy, namely, the traditionally recognised branches of learning.[6] Gāndharvaveda, Dhanurveda, Arthaśāstra and Āyurveda were recognised as *Śāstras,* i.e., the means for acquiring correct knowledge. Later on, the term *Śāstra* was used to denote any branch of study that was treated on a scientific basis. Āyurveda *Śāstra* is very vast, but the following study is only a brief survey of Āyurveda *Śāstra,* as detailed in Someśvara's Rāja Mānasollāsa.

Āyurveda or Science of Life

The Indian system of medicine called Āyurveda had its origin in the Ṛgvedic period. Rudra is spoken of as a Physician or Bhiṣak of Gods. भिषत्कमंत्वाभिषजां शृणोमि । (Ṛgveda-2.33.4). The Aśvins also are spoken of as possessing many remedies. The Atharvaveda has hymns dealing with the cure of diseases and the Purāṇas and *Smṛtis* contain accounts of medicine. Āyurveda developed in close association with the *Dharma Śāstra* and the systems of philosophy like Sāṁkhya and Yoga. The three qualities of *Prakṛti—Sattva, Rājās* and *Tamas*—are closely related to the three humours of the human body, viz., *Vāta, Pitta* and *Kapha.*

Suśruta is the author of *Suśrutasaṁhitā,* which stresses the importance of surgery. He speaks of surgical instruments and surgical operations. He must have lived around the beginning of the Christian era. Vāgbhaṭa of the 6th Century A.D., is the author of the most popular and authoritative treatise on Āyurveda known as *Aṣṭāṅgahṛdaya.* He is also the author of *Aṣṭāṅgasaṁgraha.* Nāgārjuna is the author of a treatise on Āyurveda called *Yogasāra.* The Chinese pilgrim Hieun Tsang refers to one Nāgārjuna who was an authority on Medicine and Chemistry.[7]

Indian medicine is not confined to the treatment of human beings alone. There are treatises on the treatment of animals, birds and trees. Surapāla's *Vṛkṣāyurveda,* dealing with horticulture, Nārāyaṇa's *Mātaṅgalīla* dealing with the diseases of elephants, the *Aśvāyurveda* of Gana and *Aśvacikitsā* of Jayadatta and Nakula, are some such works. The *Rājanighaṇṭu* of Narahari and *Dhanvantari Nighaṇṭu* of an unknown author are some of the *Nighaṇṭus* on the subject of Indian medicine. Someśvara mentions in Rāja Mānasollāsa the physicians who treated elephants, horses, cows, deer and birds also.[8] It can be seen that during Someśvara's period the physicians were well-versed in all types of medicines.

Definition of Āyurveda

Āyurveda consists of two words, namely, 'Āyus' and 'Veda'—meaning 'The Science of Life'. It is traditionally considered as a supplement to the Vedas. According to Caraka,[9] the question arises as to which of the four—Ṛgveda, Sāmaveda, Yajurveda, and Atharvaṇaveda do the scholars of Āyurveda follow? What is the life span? Why is it called Āyurveda? What is the object of Āyurveda? Is it eternal or ephemeral? What are its branches and how many are they? Who are eligible to study it and what for? Of the four—Ṛk, Yajus, Sāma and Atharvaṇa-Vedas, physicians owe their loyalty to the Atharvaṇa Veda because this Veda deals with diagnosis and treatment of diseases by taking recourse to gift, propitiatory rites, worship, auspicious observances, oblations, observance of spiritual rites, atonement, fast, incantations, etc. They are prescribed for the sake of longevity. Āyurveda is considered as an *Upaveda* of the Atharvaveda.

Someśvara's Rāja Mānasollāsa refers to almost all the works on Indian medicine. He uses the word *Aṣṭāṅga*[10] from Vāgbhaṭa's work, *Aṣṭāṅgahṛdaya.* This work is included in the 'Great-Trio' or '*Bṛhattrayī*'. The remaining two are *Carakasaṁhitā* by Agniveśa and the *Suśruta Saṁhitā* by Suśruta. Of these three, *Carakasaṁhitā* is considered to be the most authoritative in as much as it represents various aspects of this science, with special reference to the fundamental principles of medicine. The following *Śloka*[11] furnished towards the end of this work *(Carakasaṁhitā)* aptly describes the significance of this work. 'The methods of treatment prescribed by Agniveśa are meant both for the healthy persons (for the maintenance of their positive health and prevention of diseases) and the patients (for the cure of their ailments). Whatever is mentioned in this work may be available elsewhere and things not mentioned here are not to be found anywhere else'. This shows the importance and value of the book. In the same way, Rāja Mānasollāsa also is very important in the field of medicine. This work is useful to physicians, teachers, research workers, and students of Āyurveda.

Āyurveda has eight specialised branches. They are : (1) *Kāyacikitsā*—internal medicine, (2) *Śālākya*—treatment of diseases of the organs in the head and neck, (3) *Śalyāpahartṛka*—extraction of foreign bodies through surgery, (4) *Viṣagara-*

vairodhika-praśamana—management of conditions caused by natural and artificial poisons, (5) *Bhūtavidyā*—the treatment of psychic diseases, (6) *Kumārabhṛtya*—the treatment of children, (7) *Rasāyana*—the administration of elixirs for the maintenance of youth and prevention of old age, and lastly (8) *Vājīkaraṇa*—the administration of aphrodisiacs.[12]

Rāja Mānasollāsa also mentions eight names : *Deha, Śiras, Vāla, Viṣa, Śalya, Graha, Vṛṣya* and *Rasāyana.*[13] These names are different in the other Āyurvedic books. Vaidya Bhagwan Dash states that the names of these are : (1) Pulse, (2) Urine, (3) Stool, (4) Tongue, (5) Voice, (6) Touch (*skin*), (7) Eyes and (8) General Physical features (*Ākṛti*).[14] All these eight branches deal with the prevention and cure of diseases and morbid conditions in their respective specialised fields.

In Someśvara's Rāja Mānasollāsa, the nineteenth chapter of the first *Prakaraṇa,* deals with medical science or *Vaidyakīya-Śāstra* (1.19.135-291). He says that, for proper treatment of a disease it is essential to determine the exact nature of the disease with special reference to the *doṣas* involved. A physician must know the kind of diseases, their nature, characteristics, and so on. Further, Someśvarā mentions the qualities required in physicians.

Physicians who are born in noble families, who are well-read, who have practical experience, who are skilful and pure; whose medicinal prescriptions and surgical operations are infallible; who are self-controlled; who have all equipments and are endowed with healthy sense organs; who are acquainted with the natural symptoms; and those who have presence of mind are the saviours of life and destroyers of diseases. They are free from doubts regarding the etiology, premonitory signs and symptoms. Further he states the qualities necessary in physicians.[15] The *Caraka Saṁhitā* says that 'Excellence in medical knowledge, an extensive practical experience, dexterity and purity are the four qualities of a physician.'[16]

A person of normal mental faculty, intelligence, strength and energy, desirous of his well-being pertaining to this world and the world beyond has to satisfy three basic desires, viz., the desire to live, the desire to earn and the desire to perform virtuous acts. These three main desires belong only to such persons as are after enjoyment of happiness in this world and the world beyond. The three-fold classification of desires, therefore, does not apply to such persons to whom salvation alone is the *summum bonum* of life; nor even to such persons as have not gone above the animal instincts and so are incapable of having the three basic human desires. The desire to satisfy passions is also there, but it is in fact included under the desire to live and the desire to earn because satisfaction of passion cannot be achieved without health and wealth. For this, in fact, it is the duty of the physician to maintain the health or equilibrium of *Dhātus*. By taking recourse to concordant factors, the physician well-versed in treatment brings about equilibrium of *Dhātus* and so he is the bestower of physical happiness and longevity. Therefore, Caraka says, 'By virtue of his ability to bestow physical happiness and longevity, a physician is verily regarded as a donor of virtue, wealth and desired objects pertaining to this world and the world beyond'.[17] The states of *doṣas* in different combinations, have been explained as diseases. Hence Someśvara gives much importance to *doṣas*. He says, "*Prakṛti* or *doṣas* like *Pitta, Kapha* and *Vāta* are very important to determine diseases. Hence, a physician must take into consideration these *doṣas* or *prakṛtis* before he begins the treatment."

Someśvara has described Prakṛti as a state of life.[18] All the Hindu systems consider herbs, plants and trees as bodies endowed with life. Man is the chief among all creatures and in proportion to his complicated structure is his liability to diseases. The disorders of the human frame are of four kinds : (1) Accidental, (2) Organic, (3) Mental and (4) Natural. The injuries arising from external causes form the first class. The second comprehends the effects of the vitiated humours or derangements of the blood, bile, wind, etc. The third one is occasioned by the operation of passions, or the effects on the constitution of rage, fear, sorrow, joy, etc., and the last is referable to the necessary and innate condition of our being such as thirst, hunger, sleep, old age, and decay.

Rāja Mānasollāsa mentions some diseases like fever or *Jvara, Raktapitta, Kāsa, Śvāsa, Kṣaya, Yakṣman, Chardi Madātyaya, Arśas, Mūtrakṛchra, Prameha, Vidradhi, Śapha, Visarpa, Vātarakta,* and so on.[19] In fact, diseases are of innumerable varieties depending upon their distinctive features like pain, colour (signs), etiology (study of causes of diseases), site of origin and manifestation, symptoms (like *gulma*) and nomenclature (*rājayakṣma*) and so on. There are diseases of serious type which even though curable with difficulty, can cause death, if not treated or treated wrongly. There are other diseases of mild nature which are definitely cured by treatment. There is another category of palliable diseases which are not curable, but even the most effective treatment will only enable the patient to stand the disease. There are other diseases where no treatment can succeed. Diseases are, thus, of two types : (1) Curable and (2) incurable. Each of them is again of two types viz., mild and serious. Someśvara says, 'Sannipāta is serious but curable, only when the physician takes care in treating this disease.'[20] Further, he says that *Śopha* is incurable and serious. So hardly can any one be saved from this disease.[21]

In pre-historic times it was believed that evidences of medicine are scattered in the Vedic literature. Lord Paśupati—शिव—is regarded as the divine physician. There are many seals with his image in Harappa and Mohenjodaro. Remains of vegetable, mineral and animal substances seem to have been used in drugs. The *Oṣadhisūkta* of Ṛgveda is considered as an authentic document on ancient botany and herbaceous drugs.[22] Aśvins are considered to be endowed with remarkable healing powers and their miracles show an advanced state of medicine and surgery.[23] This seems to have developed and advanced in Atharvaveda.

Knowledge of medicine in ancient India was widespread as revealed in *Caraka Saṁhitā*, the earliest scientifically organised document on Āyurveda. *Caraka Saṁhitā* is an enlarged edition of *Agniveśatantra*. A systematic study of this work is supposed to prove how the whole system of medicine including physiology, pathology and pharmacology had been rationalised. This revolutionised the method of practising medicine in India by replacing the method of magical charms characteristic of the pre-Upaniṣadic age. The atmosphere of free thinking in the Upaniṣadic period helped in the gradual evolution of Āyurveda theories and practices.[24] The contribution of wandering mendicants or चरकs, who were experts in medicine, in this field is immense. The minute observation of nature and its phenomena has also helped in establishing the basic concepts of this science of life.

In *Aṣṭāngahṛdayam*—

आयुः कामयमानेन धर्मार्थसुखसाधनम्।
आयुर्वेदोपदेशेषु विधेयः परमादरः।। 1.2

Āyurveda has been described as a dynamic philosophy of life and not as a mere system of medicine. It is conducive to a healthy individual and social life in performing one's duty and fulfilling social obligations and attaining perfect bliss of liberation. Preservation of health in the healthy and curing illness in the diseased are stated as the twin objects of Āyurveda or science of life. Preventive medicine is given top priority in this system by giving a detailed description of daily routine keeping in mind the seasonal variations.[25]

A unique discovery of this age is described as *Lok-Purusha-Sāmānya* or the Law of Uniformity of Nature which paved the way for observation of intimate relationship between the *Purusha* and *Loka* or microcosm and macrocosm.[26]

Āyurveda regards a पुरुष—a living being as a composition of six components—पंचमहाभूतs or matter and the self or the spirit. पृथ्वी, अप्, अग्नि, वायु and आकाश are the five elements which constitute a complete human body. The outer universe has also the same material composition. So, there is similarity between the material frame of the universe and the skeleton of any living being. The self or the spirit is predominant in a human being. Every material is composed of all the पंचमहाभूतs but there is predominance of one of them according to which the organs and substances are classified in Āyurveda.

The five elements or पंचमहाभूतs only prepare the frame or the body. Only after life or after vital element enters the body, biological functions start. These functions are caused by the three vital principles known as *Vāta, Pitta* and *Kapha (sleṣma).* वात, पित्त and कफ are the three subtle forms of वायु, अग्नि (तेजस्) and अप्. In physical forms, they are represented by air, fire and water. आकाश and पृथ्वी are the remaining two भूतs. आकाश is too subtle. पृथ्वी is too gross. Both of them are not involved in the above functions.

Observation of nature and application of the Law of the Uniformity of Nature seems to have given rise to the formulation of this theory. According to Suśruta, सोम, सूर्य, वायु—(Moon, Sun, Air)—hold the cosmos by their functions of विसर्ग, आदान and विक्षेप which mean 'releasing', 'receiving' and 'disseminating'. Similarly, वात, पित्त, कफ, etc. perform these functions in a living body. सूत्रस्थान of सुश्रुतसंहिता deals with this subject in detail.

All motions, transportation and electromagnetic activities in a living body are controlled by वात. The processes of conversion, consumption and other chemical changes are caused by पित्त. कफ is concerned with water and as such maintains the body-fluid, and controls growth and strength in the body. All these exist wherever there is life and every living cell is governed by them in the performance of the functions. This is known as the theory of त्रिदोष which comprises components of प्राण—the vital element playing a predominant role in physiology and pathology. The entire living world is controlled by it. So, it applies to all the groups relating to animals—अश्वायुर्वेद, गजायुर्वेद, गवायुर्वेद and वृक्षायुर्वेद.[27]

The genetic factors are taken into account by Āyurveda. In the शरीरस्थान of चरकसंहिता, चरक has mentioned parental constituents of foetus, transference of merits and demerits including diseases and also defects in genes partially or wholly. Constitution or प्रकृति is also emphasised in Āyurveda. This considers every individual as unique and different from all others.

प्रकृति or दोषप्रकृति is determined by the preponderance of one or more दोषs at the time of fertilization.[28] For instance, if वात is predominant वातप्रकृति is characteristic of a person. Similarly, psychic constitution is determined by any of three qualities—सत्त्व, रजस् and तमस्. It is clearly mentioned in the सूत्रस्थान of चरकसंहिता that any body has to be administered only after examining the प्रकृति of each individual minutely. सुश्रुत mentions various types of physical and psychic प्रकृतिs in शरीरस्थान of सुश्रुत संहिता.

Digestion and metabolism form another important topic in आयुर्वेद. The process of conversion of ingested substances into assimilable form is known as digestion. This process is governed by अग्नि known as जठराग्नि as this is situated in जठर or abdomen. The process of digestion is governed by the digestive fire which consists of various juices. Without its proper functioning, assimilation of food is not possible. Without अग्नि no transformation or conversion can take place. In the चिकित्सास्थान of चरकसंहिता there is an elaborate description of this digestion process of food consumed.

The work Rāja Mānasollāsa has paid great attention to

regimen (prescribed diet and habits). Someśvara opines that food is not digested by a patient suffering from fever. So for him, the physician must start treatment with regulation of diet.[29]

He gives a number of rules relating to food and describes the general treatment, suited to the complaint or favourable to the operation of medicine administered. This branch in the Rāja Mānasollāsa is entitled *Abhakṣavarjana.* Some other books call it *Pathyāpathya.* To these subjects are to be added the *Cikitsā,* or medical treatment of diseases, on which subject, there are a variety of compositions, which contain much that is of value.

Someśvara explains what is meant by *Laṅghana* or diet control. He says, "Do not take the food of these five types, namely, *Bhakṣya,* to be chewed by teeth, *Bhojya* to be taken without chewing, *Coṣya* to suck, *Lehya* to lick and *Peya* to drink". It is called *Laṅghana.* This is the first preparation for the medical treatment.[30] Further he tells, "A physician must know the age of the patient, and *Vāta, Pitta* and *Kapha's* strength and strength of the patient, time, *prakṛti,* and *Nidāna* before the starting of *Laṅghana.* This *Laṅghana* is continued till the body is purified".[31] Someśvara says that this *Laṅghana* is of many varieties, according to the *Doṣas.*[32] It has been already mentioned that food is most important in medical treatment. Modern physicians also give much importance to food. In modern science, food articles are primarily classified depending upon their chemical composition, namely, carbohydrates, proteins, fats, vitamins, minerals, etc. In Rāja Mānasollāsa, such classification is based on the biological action of the food articles and their *Rasa* (taste). Someśvara mentions many varieties of food, its preparation, and so on. All varieties of rice may be treated as of one group on the basis of their carbohydrate content. But Āyurveda considers that freshly harvested rice is heavy for digestion. It aggravates *Kapha.* If used continuously, it is supposed to produce many complications. Old rice stored for over six months is considered to be light and more useful for an average person. The freshly harvested rice produces more fat in the body, than the old rice. Thus, for an emaciated individual having good digestive power, freshly harvested rice is nutritious, whereas for a fat person, even without good digestive power, old rice is nutritious. Pulses contain mostly protein. But according to Āyurveda, some of them like *Māṣa* (black gram) is heavy for digestion as it produces more fat in the body whereas *Mudga* (green gram) is considered to be light for digestion and it reduces fat in the body. *Kulattha* on the other hand, is exceedingly nutritious for fat persons. Mild fire should be used for cooking the pulses. Someśvara says that horse gram and green gram should be cooked on mild fire.[33]

Āyurveda considers mental power as very important. Mental activities are more powerful than the physical activities. *Manas* is the controller of the body. Āyurveda in general, and Rāja Mānasollāsa in particular, attach considerable importance to the intimate relationship between the mind (mental activities) and the body (physical functions). Any disturbance in the one, affects the other and causes diseases. Therefore, both for maintaining positive health as well as for curing of diseases, both the mind and the body are required to be kept in proper condition. *Utsāha* is important in all types of functions.[34] *Utsāha* means enthusiasm. Someśvara himself tells, "The person, who has no mental worries is the only healthy person. His actions always give fruits. He is fit for the *gītagosthi* and other entertainment."[35]

According to Vaidya Bhagwan Dash, "The concept of mind is very important and significant to both Āyurveda and Yoga. In Āyurveda, diseases are classified into two categories, viz., Physical and Mental. In the former, the body is considered to be the seat of the disease and in the latter, the mind. In both categories, the mind plays an important role in causing diseases. Psychic factors exercise control over the physiological functions of the body and vice versa. Therefore, even for the treatment of some physical diseases certain psychic measures are prescribed in Āyurveda.[36] Caraka says that physical exercises are helpful for health.[37] Further, Caraka tells : 'The virtuous one, who is free from all vices relating to mind, speech and physical actions, is indeed happy and he alone enjoys the fruits of virtues (*Dharma*), wealth (*Artha*) and desire (*Kāma*).[38] Mental conditions like worry, grief, fear and anger are described as causative factors for indigestion even if wholesome food is taken in proper quantity. Someśvara has, in the Mānasōllasa, a separate *Prakaraṇa* relating to seasonal entertainments and games, for the maintenance of health. There is the proverb that "Health is wealth". Kālidāsa says in his *Kumārasaṁbhava* that 'body is the best means for practising *Dharma*'.[39]

The Rāja Mānasollāsa mentions the names of a few diseases. It tells how to control diseases as per the rules and regulation of the *Vaidyaśāstra.* Someśvara suggests that diseases should be counteracted according to *Vaidyaśāstra.*[40] For the proper treatment of diseases, it is essential to determine the exact nature of the disease with special reference to the *Doṣas, Dhātus, Malas, Srotas,* and *Agnis* involved in its manifestation. Āyurvedic classics impress upon the physician not to be very particular about the name of the disease. According to these classics, names are attributed to some of these diseases only by way of example to facilitate the physician to ascertain and understand the details of the remaining diseases. In respect of each disease, whether named or unnamed, the physicians' careful examination is needed.

The basic elements of the body are known as *Dhātus* in all the texts of the *Āyurvedaśāstra.* "The *Dhātu,* etymologically means, one which assists the body or which enters into the formation of the basic structure of the body as a whole."[41] These *Dhātus* are seven in number and they are : (1) *Rasa,* (2) *Rakta,* (3) *Māṁsa,* (4) *Medas,* (5) *Asthi,* (6) *Majja* and (7) *Śukra.* According to Vaidya Bhagwan Dash, "These seven *Dhātus* are composed of the five *Mahābhūtas. Pṛthvi-Mahābhūta* predominates the muscle and fat tissues. *Jala-Mahābhūta* predominates the lymph and chyle. The haemoglobin fraction of the blood is primarily constituted of *Tejas-Mahābhūta.* The bone is composed of *Vāyu-Mahābhūta* and the pores inside the bones are dominated by *Ākāśa-Mahābhūta.* It should be made clear again that all the seven *Dhātus* are composed of all the five *Mahābhūtas* and only the dominating *Mahābhūtas* are described above. These *Dhātus* remain inside the human body of the individual in a particular proportion, and any change in their equilibrium leads to disease and decay".[42] The *Doṣas* in the body are composed of five *Mahābhūtas,* i.e.,

1. *Kapha* is dominated by *Pṛthvi* and *Jala;*
2. *Pitta* is dominated by *Agni;*
3. *Vāyu* is dominated by *Vāyu* and *Ākāśa.*

Hence, a drug is composed of five *Mahābhūtas,* namely, *Ākāśa, Vāyu, Tejas, Jala and Pṛthvi.*[43] Someśvara has stated that a physician must treat after knowing all the factors, namely, strong, middle, and low diseases, place, time, age and the condition of the patient.[44] Someśvara further tells about a good physician. "He who clearly knows the causes and the names of the diseases, and the names and characteristics of medicines, is the best physician."[45]

Sapta Dhātus

These constitute the supporting structure of the body. They are :

1. रस — *Rasa* .... the primary product of food-digestion.
2. रक्त — *Rakta* .... blood.
3. मांस — *Māmsa* .... flesh-muscles and tendons.
4. मेदस् — *Medas* ... fat.
5. अस्थिन् — *Asthin* .... bone.
6. मज्जन् — *Majjan* .... bone-marrow.
7. शुक्रम् — *Śukram* .... vital fluid.

These are called '*dūṣya*'—दूष्य also, as they are liable to be vitiated by the *tridoṣas* in their pathogenic state. They represent, to some extent, the connective and nervous tissues of modern physiology. In them are to be found the *tridoṣas* in their normal gross forms. They are said to inherit also the *guṇās* of the *Panca-mahābhūtas.* The following quotation from Dalhaṇa's commentary supports this statement[46] :

The functions of the *Sapta-dhātus* : The functions of the *Sapta-dhātus* in their normal condition are as follows :

1. *Rasa* gives a feeling of satisfaction (प्रीणन) and promotes the formation of blood.
2. *Rakta*—is enlivening or life-giving (जीवन); contributes to a healthy complexion (वर्णप्रसादन) and leads to the formation of मांसधातु.
3. *Mansa*—contributes to the fullness (nourishment) of the body (शरीरपुष्टि) and produces *Medas.*
4. *Medas*—gives oiliness and warmth to the body (*Snehana*), imparts firmness and stability to the bones and helps their growth.
5. *Asthin*—supports the body (धारण) and promotes the formation of *Majjan.*
6. *Majjan*—fills up the interior portions of bones (पूरण), gives strength to the body, creates affection and attachment, and nourishes *Śukram.*
7. *Śukram*—accomplishes the purpose of emission, bestows courage and strength, creates attraction for the opposite sex and pleasure in their company, and is responsible for conception and reproduction (गर्भोत्पादन).

ओजस् is the quintessence of all the *dhātus.* Its main locus is the heart (हृदय), though it is true that it pervades the whole body.

Its properties and functions are described below :

ओजः सोमातत्मकं स्निग्धं शुक्लं शीतं स्थिरं सरम्।
विविक्तं मृदु मृत्स्नं च प्राणायतनमुत्तमम्।।
देहस्यावयवस्तेन व्याप्तो भवति देहिनाम्।
तदभावाच्च शीर्यन्ते शरीराणि शरीरिणाम्।।

(चरकसंहिता-सूत्रस्थान 15.25-26)

It is responsible for the maintenance and upkeep of the body. When it perishes, the body is invariably destroyed, and life exists so long as it is expected to; the various activities, functions and features of the system are entirely dependent on it.

Nourishment of the *Sapta-Dhātus* by *Āhāra-rasa*

Rasa—'त्रिधातुसमुदायात्मक आहाररसः'—is the essence of the food ingested and digested properly. It gets circulated to all parts of the body through the lymphatics and the blood-vessels, nourishes and supports them and helps their development. Its situation is the heart, because, it comes back to the heart after being driven from it to all the parts, and playing its part in the nutritional functions. It is *Pañca-bhautika* in character as it is the essence of *Āhāra-dravyas*. Suśruta says,[47] "it is endowed with potential heat obtained during the digestive processes". So, it imparts its *Pañca-bhautika* character to all the seven *dhātus*. It is, therefore, called पोषकरस, a name distinguished from पोष्यरस applied to the आद्यधातु, the first of the seven *dhātus*. Suśruta and Caraka support this view in the following words :

(रसः) स तु व्यानेन विक्षिप्तः सर्वान् धातून् प्रतर्पयेत्।।

(सुश्रुतसंहिता-सूत्रस्थान 46.426)

व्यानेन रसधातुर्हि विक्षेपोचितकर्मणा।
युगपत् सर्वतोऽजस्त्रं देहे विक्षिप्यते सदा।।

(चरकसंहिता-चिकित्सा 15.35)

It can very well be inferred from these quotations that *Rasa-dhātu* plays the same part in circulation as the blood in modern physiology. The nerves which impel the circulation are contained in *Vyāna-vāyu* which is supplied to all the parts of the body and is also closely connected with vasomotor systems.

In this connection Suśruta says[48]—

The sum and substance of these verses as stated earlier is that, *Anna-rasa* (अन्नरस) gives nourishing material to the tissues, both directly and indirectly. The direct method is the one explained by the general statement "सर्वदा सर्वभावानाम् सामान्यं वृद्धिकारणम्।" The indirect nourishment is conducted stage by stage through the processes of analysis and synthesis in *dhātu*-formation. The *Pañcha-bhautika Āhāra* consisting of the *Ṣadrasas* nourishes the *Tridhātus*. Then the *Tridhātus* nourish the *Saptadhātus*. The *Ādya-dhātu-rasa* (आद्यधातुरस) requires to be enriched with pigment before it is converted into blood. It gets its share of pigment—haemoglobin—from the liver and the spleen, when it passes through them. This haemoglobin is a by-product of 'ferratin'—an iron containing body stored up in the liver. Further, as the process of development goes on, *Māmsa* (मांस) is nourished by *Rakta* (रक्त), *Medas* (मेदस्), by *Māmsa, Asthin* (अस्थिन्) by *Medas, Majjan* (मज्जन) by *Asthin* and *Śukram* (शुक्रम्) by *Majjan*. These processes are brought about chiefly by Agni. Caraka says :

यदन्नं देहधात्वोजोबलवर्णादि पोषकम्।
तत्राग्निर्हेतुराहारान्न ह्यपक्वाद्रसादयः।।

(चरकसंहिता-चिकित्सा 5.4)

The nutritional value of food which nourishes the body, its tissues, vital essence ओजस्, strength, complexion etc., is mainly dependent on Agni; because *Rasa* and other *dhātus* cannot develop from undigested food.

Agni in the form of *Pitta-dhātu* is present everywhere in the body and in consequence of this a constant process of 'digestion' is going on in every part of the body. *Agni* implied here is both of a potential as well as of a kinetic type. In this connection the Āyurvedists have mentioned thirteen kinds of Agni. They are—

1. The seven धात्वग्निs—*Agnis* existing in the *Sapta-dhātus* and their सूक्ष्मावयवs, the cells.
2. The five भूताग्निs—which belong to the *pañcha mahābhūtas.*
3. जठराग्नि—the heat produced in the digestive processes in the gastro-intestinal tract.

Of these *agnis,* the one with the gastro-intestinal origin is the most important. For, upon the variations of this digestive heat depends the वृद्धि and क्षय of both भूताग्नि and धात्वग्नि. (Vide verses 36 and 37, *Chikitsasthāna,* Ch. 15, Caraka). This heat breaks up the compactness of food and reduces it, by analysis into similar substances. Caraka clearly opines that[49]—

The five *agnis* belonging to the five elements operate upon the five elemental portions of *Āhāra-dravya* (आहारद्रव्य) with the result that शब्द, स्पर्श, रूप, रस and गन्ध are exhibited in the body-tissues. As the *gunās* of the *Pañcabhūtas* are transferred to *Saptadhātus,* the धात्वग्निs belonging to the latter behave in a similar way. In this way, the *Pañchabhautika* properties शब्दादिगुण of food nourish the corresponding *Pañchabhautika* properties of the body-content.

Analysis and Synthesis in *Dhātu* formation

When the *Saptadhātus* are being thus nourished, each with its own *agni,* certain processes of analysis and synthesis take place in their constituents. Each of these *dhātus* is broken up into three sets of products. *Śukra,* the last one, is an exception as it has no *Mala* in a healthy condition. One of these sets (by-products) contributes to the growth of the स्थायीधातु, the second—सूक्ष्म—contributes to the next tissue (*dhātu*) in order and the third takes part in the *Mala-dhātu.* This is expressed in the following lines :

स्थूलसूक्ष्ममलैः सर्वे भिद्यन्ते धातवस्त्रिधा।
स्वः स्थूलोंऽशः परं सूक्ष्मस्तन्मलं याति तन्मलः।।
स्वाग्निभिः पच्यमानेषु मलः षट्सु रसादिषु।
न शुक्रे पच्यमानेऽपि हेमनीवाक्षये मलः।।

(सुश्रुतसंहिता-सूत्रस्थान 14.10)

The *Malas* of the different *dhātus* produced after digestion (action and reaction), referred to above are :

किट्टमन्नस्य विण्मूत्रं रसस्य तु कफोऽस्त्रजः।।
पित्तं मांसस्य च मलो मलः खेदस्तु मेदसः।
स्यात्किट्टं केशलोमाऽस्थ्नो मज्जः स्नेहोऽक्षिविट् त्वचाम्।।
प्रसादकिट्टे धातूनां पाकादेवंविधःस्मृतः।
परस्परोपसंस्तंभाधातुस्नेहपरंपरा।।

(चरकसंहिता-चिकित्सा 15.29-30)

In the last line of the above quoted *Śloka* we see, "Such is the force of heredity manifested in the adjustment of stability and mutual co-operation among the tissue-elements by a process of interaction." These views of the Āyurvedic writers regarding the developmental (natural tendencies) proclivities of the tissues and their elementary parts point out clearly that the concept entertained by them is not imaginary. The interdependence of the tissue-elements exhibited in the maintenance of the balance of life through the influence of their by-products, प्रसादाख्य or मलाख्य, suggests that the supersensory (अतीन्द्रिय) processes are conducted through a mechanism other than the Central Nervous System. This mechanism is nothing but the influence of the *Tridoṣas* in their subtle state, actuated by the intrinsic faculties of अध्यामगुणसंग्रह.

शरीरावयवास्तु परिमाणुभेदेनापरिसंख्येया भवन्त्यतिबहुत्वादतिसौक्ष्म्यादतीन्द्रियत्वाच्च, तेषां संयोगविभागे परमाणूनां कारणं वायुः कर्म स्वभावश्च।। 16।।

(चरकसंहिता-चिकित्सा 7.16)

It cannot be denied that there is, in health, a sort of organic equilibrium between cellular elements of the different tissues and the products of their secretion. It may, therefore, be concluded that the alterations which affect certain alimentary cells in the body always react on the corresponding anatomical elements, and modify the constitution of their structure.

The interchange of matter secreted by these cellular groups is more intrinsic and contributes to the primary stages of development in organic evolution. The line 'स्वस्थूलोऽश: परं सूक्ष्मस्तन्मलं याति तन्मल:' goes to show how the nourishment of different tissues रस:, रक्त, मांस, मेदस्, अस्थिन्, मज्जन् and शुक्र is maintained in a certain order of progression from *Rasa* onwards, each सूक्ष्म portion influencing the structure of the next *dhātu* in the course of development. The order of succession in the developmental process indicates how complex bodies are formed from simple ones, how the interchange of internal secretions (not necessarily endocrines) pertaining to the cellular groups become thicker as developments proceeds, and how nature, irrespective of any definite propensities (inclinations), adapts itself to conditions in the development of the organism.

These statements can be verified by some pathological facts, e.g., if *Madhura-rasa* (मधुररस), which is consumed with the food, is larger in proportion than the quantity required, *Medas-dhātu* is developed. In this connection Suśruta says[50]—

Growth, in fact, is an exceedingly complex process due to multitudinous factors, and we cannot give priority in importance to one over the other, as all of them are working in co-operation with one another.

Sometimes, king Someśvara uses the words *sitaih śāstraiḥ,*[51] which refer to sharp instruments. At the time of Someśvara, the physicians knew the surgical science also. Further, the Rāja Mānasollāsa discusses various aspects of medical treatment such as *Yantras,* i.e., implements, *Śastras,* i.e., instruments, *agni,* i.e., fire, *Śalākā,* i.e., pins or thin bars, *Śṛṅga,* i.e., the horns of animals and so on (1.19. 285-288). The subsidiary means are *Nīrajā* i.e., leeches.[52]

Other supplementary articles required in surgery are *Kṣāra* i.e., alkaline or alkalescent salts. Someśvara's Rāja Mānasollāsa tells us about the preparation of various types of *Kṣāra*. Someśvara directs the physician to know the characteristics of *Vāta, Pitta* and *Kapha* and then to give *Kaṣāya. Kaṣāya* is obtained by burning different herbal substances, i.e., *Vanaspatis,* and *Dravyas,* and boiling the ashes with five or six times measure of water. These *Kaṣāyas* cure the particular diseases. In some cases the concentrated solution is used after straining, and is administered orally, as well as applied externally.[53]

For the latter purpose, however, Śārṅgadhara directs the solution, after straining, to be boiled to dryness by which, of course, a carbonate of potash will be obtained, more or less caustic according to its purity. It is not unlikely that some of the herbal substances used will yield a tolerably pure alkali. Care is enjoined in their use. At the same time these and the other substitutes have to be employed where it is necessary to humour the weakness of the patient. Hence, Someśvara says, "Good medicines, *Kaṣāyas,* or drugs are similar to Nectar."[54] Drugs and diet having six tastes are wholesome to the body and as such they add to the growth of blood, muscle, fat, bone marrow, semen and longevity.

The Vedas and *Dharmaśāstra* prescribe various remedies for the people who are suffering from multiple diseases caused by their sins committed knowingly or unknowingly in the same birth or in the previous births. Someśvara states that *Krūra Karma* is a cause for disease. As stated earlier, a king is enjoined to look after his subjects as his own children, as per the dictates of *Rājadharma.* The basic tenets of *Rajadharma* are the observances of *Japa, Tapa, Vṛta, Niyama,* etc. This will ensure peace of mind. Ancient Indian works specifically recommend that, "*Dāna, Japa, Homa, Vrata,* etc., are better remedies than medicines, since *Dāna, Japa* etc., are not only capable of curing the diseases but also powerful in destroying the root cause, viz., sins."[55]

Someśvara clearly says, "If a person follows the rules of *Brahmacarya* and practises *Tapa, Indriyanigraha, Japa, Dhyāna, Prāṇāyāma, Samādhi* and *Niyamas,* he gets even the difficult desires fulfilled."[56]

It is only after digestion, आहाररस (essence of food), is absorbed and carried into the circulation of blood. आहाररस is absorbed into रसधातु already existing in the blood.[57] आहाररस is known as पोषकरस and रसधातु is known as पोष्यरस। धातुs are supporting tissues and entities. They are seven in number as already mentioned. They are all formed by their respective अग्निs. Activation of अग्नि produces essence and excrement. Essence is आहाररस and the excrement is faeces and urine. At the level of metabolism or धातुपाक, the two portions become quite distinct.

Besides, अग्निस्रोतम् or channels, also play an important role in this process. रस traverses in the body through channels as water flows in irrigating channels in the field.[58]

Āyurveda holds ओजस् as an important component in a living being. ओजस् is considered as the essence of all धातुs. ओजस् is neither धातु nor उपधातु, but has an independent position.[59] ओजस् is said to be seated in हृदय and intimately connected with प्राण. Non-living beings can survive without ओजस्. ओजस् is described as of two types. परा—superior and अपरा—inferior. The affection of the latter causes various symptoms, whereas the former causes death. ओजक्षय or dimunition of ओजस् causes many disorders; even death.

Regulation and control of diet forms a very important chapter in चरकसंहिता. The nutritive value and the digestibility have to be kept in mind while prescribing any diet. Quantum of food is also given due prominence. चरकसंहिता deals exhaustively in सूत्रस्थान (5-12) about a balanced diet. Diet also nourishes the mind and as such one has to be very careful in selecting items suited to mental qualities.[60] This subject is discussed at several places in Mānasollāsa also.

Āyurveda gives special importance to प्रकृतिस्थापना—restoration of normalcy which is the main object of a physician. प्रकृति is normalcy or equilibrium, whereas विकृति is disorder or disequilibrium. Equilibrium of psychosomatic elements is health and its absence is disease. Health is maintained by avoiding extremes and following a middle path. साम्य is equilibrium and वैषम्य is disequilibrium. समयोग is the result of साम्य which is necessary for health. अयोग, (non-use); अतियोग (excessive use) and मिथ्यायोग (faulty use) cause वैषम्य resulting in disease.[61] Maintenance of health of the healthy person and restoration of the health of diseased person is the main object of a physician.

In modern times chemistry is considered the basis of drug composition. In Āyurveda पंचमहाभूतs constitute the basis of the composition of drugs or द्रव्यs.

Every drug in Āyurveda is पंचमहाभौतिक.[62] Each material substance can be used as a drug as it is composed of पंचमहाभूतs.[63] Every drug has some qualities and actions.[64] Drugs are mostly inferred by *Rasas* or tastes. *Rasas* are the result of पंचभौतिक composition of the drug. These drugs have effects on दोषs. मधुर—sweet, आम्ल—sour, लवण—salty, कटु—Pungent, तिक्त—bitter and कषाय—astringent are six *Rasas*. They influence दोषs. *Rasas* have their own actions. Excessive use of the *Rasas* causes disorder.[65]

Chemistry was known to the people in ancient India. Chemicals and medicines were hand-made. Chemists apparently devoted most of their attention to making medicines and drugs to promote health and longevity. According to D.D. Mehta "Chemistry is a branch of Medicine."[66] Beginning from the references to medicine in the Ṛgveda[67] and Atharvaveda,[68] we can trace an unbroken continuity of medical tradition. From them, we come to know that there were hundreds of medical practitioners and thousands of medicines, prepared from herbs and plants. The Ṛgveda[69] refers to the functions of a physician. From these references we can infer that in the Vedic period, medical tradition consisted of a large number of physicians and medicines.

In the Ṛgveda, the Aśvins are the heavenly physicians. Their medical and surgical achievements are many and varied—

दीर्घतमा मामतेयो जुजुर्वान् दशमे युगे।
अपामर्थं यतीनां ब्रह्मा भवति सारथिः।। (1.158.6)

and to them are offered prayers for giving medicine—

शतमिन्नु शरदो अन्ति देवा यत्रा नश्चक्रा जरसं तनूनाम्।
पुत्रासो यत्र पितरो भवन्ति मा नो मध्या रिरीषतायुर्गन्तोः।।
(1.89.9)

They possess great knowledge of plants and herbs; they, by their power, give strength to limbs, remove old age and grant long life—

प्र वां दंसांस्यश्विनाववोचमस्य पतिः स्यां सुगवः सुवीरः।
उत पश्यन्नश्नुवन् दीर्घमायुरस्तमिवेज्जरिमाणं जगम्याम्।।
(1.116.25)

Rudra is the first heavenly physician[70] and the best among the physicians.[71] In the Ṛgveda Rudra's medicines are mentioned many times.

Someśvara has included all types of knowledge in the Rāja Mānasollāsa. First of all, he shows that he was a follower of the ancestors in the field of *Rasāyana* or Chemistry. He divides *Rasāyana* into two types, namely, *Kuṭipraveśana* and second *Vātātapasaha*.[72] Preparation of all types of medicines in the house is called *Kuṭipraveśana Rasāyana*. And the preparation of all types of medicines in the open ground is called the *Vātātapasaha*. A king has to undertake many works, such as executive work, administrative work, and judicial work. So, for the king *Vātātapasaha Rasāyana* is preferred. Someśvara knew the art of preparation of medicines from herbs,[73] fruits,[74] food-grains[75] and so on. He also wishes that a king should have a sound health and long life. This will enable him to discharge his duties and responsibilities towards himself and his subjects effectively.

तस्माद् रसायनान् योगान् यत्नान् सेवेत पार्थिवः।
दृढगात्रो भवेत् तेन वलीपतिलवर्जितः।।
जीवेच्च सुचिरं कालं राजा रोगविवर्जितः।
तस्माद् रसायनं वक्ष्ये नृपाणां हितकाम्यया।।

(2.1.12-13)

References

1. ब्रह्मणा हि यथाप्रोक्तमायुर्वेदं प्रजापतिः।... *Caraka Saṁhitā—Sūtrasthāna* 1.4.24.
2. इह खल्वायुर्वेदं... श्लोकशतसहस्रमध्यायसहस्रं च कृतवान् स्वयम्भूः।
Suśruta Saṁhitā—Sūtrasthāna 1.6.
3. *Kaśyapa Saṁhitā* 6.1.10.
4. K.G. Zysk, *Asceticism and healing in ancient India* (Oxford University Press, New York and Oxford, 1991), pp. 17-99.
5. T.K. Ramachandra Iyer, *A Short History of Sanskrit Literature* (R.S. Vedhyar and Sons, Book-sellers and Publishers, Kalpathi 1997). pp. 55-100.
Cf. also W.K. Lele. *The Doctrine of the Tantrayuktis*, Chaukhamba Surabharati Prakashan, Varanasi, 1981).
M.S. Sastry. *Sanskrita Kavi Jivitam* Ed. by P. Sri Ramachandradu and V. Sundara Sarma (Sanskrit Academy, Osmania University, Hyderabad, 1982).
6. अङ्गानि षट् वेदाश्चत्वारो मीमांसान्यायविस्तरः।
पुराणं धर्मशास्त्रं च विद्याह्येताश्चतुर्दश। T.K. Ramachandra Iyer, *op.cit.*, p. 98.
7. T.K. Ramachandra Iyer, *op.cit.*, p. 171.
8. नराणां च गजानां च वाजिनां च गवामपि।
मृगाणां च खगानां च ये जानन्ति चिकित्सितम्।। (2.2.138)
9. तत्र चेत् प्रष्टारः स्युः चतुर्णामृक्सामयजुरथर्व-वेदानां कं वेदमुपदिशन्त्यायुर्वेदविदः? किमायुः? कस्मादायुर्वेदः? किमर्थमायुर्वेदः? शाश्वतोऽशाश्वतो? कति कानि चास्याङ्गानि? कैश्चायमध्येतव्यः? किमर्थं च इति।
तत्र भिषजा पुष्टेनैवं चतुर्णामृक्सामयजुरथर्व वेदानामात्मनोऽथर्ववेदभक्तिरादेश्यास्या। वेदो ह्यथर्वणो दानस्वस्त्ययनवलिमङ्गलहोमनियमप्रायश्चित्तोपवासमन्त्रादिपरिग्रहा च्चिकित्सा प्राहं, चिकित्सा चायुषो हितायोपदिश्यते।। (चरकसंहिता 30.20.21)
10. परं पारङ्गताः सम्यगष्टाङ्गेतु चिकित्सिते।
शस्त्रकर्मकलादधा मन्त्रे तन्त्रे च कोविदाः।। (2.2.139)

11. चिकित्सा वह्निवेशस्य सुस्थानुरहितं प्रति।
यदिहास्ति तदन्यत्र यन्नेहास्ति न तत्क्वचित्।। (चरकसंहिता-सिद्धिस्थान 12.53-54)
12. तस्यायुर्वेदस्याङ्गान्यष्टौ, तथा–कायचिकित्सा, शालाक्यं, शल्यापहर्तृकं, विषगरवैरोधिकप्रशमनं, भूतविद्या, कौमारभृत्यकं, रसायनं, वाजिकरणमिति।। (तदेव 30.28)
13. देहे शिरसि बाले तु चिषे शल्ये ग्रहेऽपि च।
वृष्ये रसायने चैव कुशला भिषजोऽष्टसु।। (2.20.340)
14. Vaidya Bhagwan Dash. *Fundamentals of Āyurvedic Medicine* IIIrd Vol. (Bansal and Co., New Delhi, 1982), p. 93.
15. शस्त्र-शास्त्रविदो वैद्यानभ्यासनिपुणानपि।
ऊहापोहविवेकज्ञान् सुदाहस्तान् प्रियंवदान्।। (1.19.139)
16. श्रुते पर्यवदातत्वं बहुशो दृष्टकर्मता।
दाक्ष्यं शौधमिति ज्ञेयं वैद्ये गुणमतुष्टकम्।। (चरकसंहिता-सूत्रस्थान 9.6)
17. धर्मस्यार्थस्य कामस्य नृलोकस्योभयस्य च।
दाता संपद्यते वैद्यो दानाद् देहसुसायुषाम्।। (*Ibid.*, सूत्रस्थान-38)
18. ज्ञात्वा निदानं व्याधीनां स्वरूपं लक्षणैः स्फुटम्।
देशकालानुसारेण सात्म्यप्रकृतितत्त्वतः।। (1.19.144)
19. ज्वरे च रक्तपित्ते च कासेश्वासे च यक्ष्मणि।
छर्दौ मदात्ययेऽर्शःसु सारण ग्रहणीषु च।।
मूत्रकृच्छ्रे प्रमेहे च विद्रधौ गुल्म-कोष्ठयोः।
पाण्डौ शोके विसर्पे च कृष्णे शिवत्रे बलामये।।
वातशोणितरोगे च तथा रोगान्तरेष्वपि।
वैद्यशास्त्रानुसारेण कारयेत् तत्प्रतिक्रियाम्।। (1.19.141-143)
20. दोषत्रय-प्रकुपिते सन्निपातो भवेत् समे।
दुश्चिकित्सो भवेद् रोगी यत्नादेनमुपाचरेत्।। (1.19.159)
21. सन्निपातज्वरान्मुक्ते शोफो भवति दारुणः।
कर्णमूले यदा तेन कश्चिदेव विमुच्यते।। (1.19.198)
22. *Ṛg Veda.* 1.181.1-8; 8.47.1-14; 10.40.1-14; 10.34.1-14.
23. आयुर्वेद का वैज्ञानिक इतिहास, प्रियव्रतशर्मा, पृ० 13, 17.
24. P.V. Sharma, 'Dr. P.M. Mehta Memorial Lecture', Jamnagar, 1989.
25. *Ibid.*
26. सोऽयमायुर्वेदः शाश्वतो निर्दिश्यते, अनादित्वात्, स्वभावसंसिद्धलक्षणत्वात्, भावस्वभावनित्यत्वाच्च। (चरकसंहिता-सूत्रस्थान 30-27)
27. प्रियव्रतशर्मा, *op.cit.*, p. 64.
28. शुक्रशोणितसंयोगे यो भवेद्दोष उत्कटः।
प्रकृतिर्जायते तेन तस्या मे लक्षणं शृणु।। (सुश्रुत संहिता-शरीरस्थान 4.63)
29. अजीर्यत्याषर्थं यस्याज्ज्वरार्तस्य विनाऽग्निना।
तस्मान्न दमाद् भेषज्यं लङ्घनं तु प्रयोजयेत्।। (1.19.148)

30. भक्ष्यभोज्यस्य चोष्यस्य लेह्य-पेयस्य वारणम्।
लङ्घनं प्रोच्यते सद्भिः कायलाघवकारणम्।। (1.19.149)
31. वायोदोषं बलं कालं प्रकृतिं कारणं तथा।
विचार्य लङ्घनं कार्यं यावच्छुद्धं भवेद् वपुः।। (1.19.150)
32. एकभक्तं तथा पेया मण्डो वा कोष्णवारिवा।
दोषकोपानुसारेण लङ्घनं विविधं स्मृतम्।। 1.19.153)
33. प्रक्षालितान् वरान् मुद्गन् समतोये विनिक्षिपेत्।
चुल्यां मृद्वग्निना पाकः कर्तव्यः सूपकारकः।।
द्विथरः पूर्षवत् कार्यः पाकः पाकविचक्षणैः।
पच्यमाने षुमुद्गेषु हिङ्गुचारि विनिक्षिपेत्।। (3.13.1367-68)
34. प्रारब्धं यत् स्वयं कार्यं दैवाद् यदि न सिध्यति।
न सीदति च तत् कर्तुमुत्साही च पुनः पुनः।।
यस्य स्यादुद्यमे नित्यं चित्तमुत्साह-संयुतम्।
उत्साहशक्तिः सा ज्ञेया नृपाणां भूतिमिच्छताम्।। (2.2.723-24)
35. भूलोकमल्लदेवेन कथ्यते गीतसंश्रयः।
नीरूजः स्वस्थचित्तश्च कृतकार्यो महाघनः।।
तृप्तो हृष्टमना गीते विनोदं कर्तुमर्हति।
शृङ्गारी दानशूरश्च सर्वशास्त्रार्थतत्वचित्।। (4.16.1.2)
36. Vaidya Bhagwan Dash, *Fundamentals of Āyurvedic Medicine* (Bansal and Co., Delhi, IIIrd ed., 1982), p. 49.
37. शरीरचेष्टा या चेष्टा स्थैर्यार्थबलवर्धिनी।
देहव्यायामसंख्याता मात्रया तां समाचरेत्।। (चरकसंहिता सूत्रस्थान 7.31)
38. पुण्यशब्दो विपाकत्वान्मनोवाक्कायकर्मणाम्।
धर्मार्थकामान् पुरुषः सुखी भुङ्क्ते चिनोति च।। (तदेवं 7.30)
39. शरीरमाद्यं खलु धर्म-साधनम्। (कालिदास, कुमारसंभव, सर्ग 5)
40. वैद्यशास्त्रानुसारेण कारयेत् तत्प्रतिक्रियाम्। (1.19.143)
41. विकारो धातुवैषम्यं, साम्यं प्रकृतिरुच्यते।
सुखसंज्ञकमारोग्यं, विकारो दुःखमेव च।। (चरक संहिता सूत्रस्थान 9.4)
42. Vaidya Bhagwan Dash, *op.cit.*, p. 28.
43. *Ibid.*, p. 59.
44. कृच्छसाध्यमसाध्यं वा साध्यं जानन्ति तत्त्वतः।
देशं कालं वयोऽवस्थां प्रकृतिसात्म्यमेव च।। (2.3.114)
45. रोगनामनिदानं तु रुजं जानन्ति तत्त्वतः।
औषधं रूप-नामभ्यां जानन्तो भिषजो वराः।। (2.2.141)
46. यद्यापि पंचभूतानां वाच्यः पाको द्विधा पुनः।
तथाप्यपां प्रधानत्वाद्रसः सौम्योऽभिधीयते।।
अतिरिक्ता गुणा रक्ते वन्हेर्मांसे तु पार्थिवाः।

मेदस्यम्बुभुवोरस्थ्नि पृथिव्यनिलतेजसाम्।
मज्ज्ञि शुक्रे वा सौम्यस्य मूत्रेऽम्बुशिखिनोर्गुणा।
भुवो विश्यार्तवे त्वग्ने: प्रस्वेदस्तन्ययोरपाम्।।
इति धातुमलेषूक्ता गुणा: प्रधान्यत: स्थिता:।
प्रायेण भूगुणा गर्भे स्तोकाद्यनुग्रहा इति।। (सुश्रुतसंहिता-सूत्रस्थान 15.1-4)

47. पंचभूतात्मके देहे आहार: पांचभौतिक:।
विपक्व: पंचधा सम्यग्गुणान् स्वानभिवर्धयेत्।। (सुश्रुतसंहिता-सूत्रस्थान 46.524)

48. स खलु आप्यो रसो यकृत्प्लीहानौ प्राप्य रागमुपैति।।
रंजितास्तेजसा त्वाप: शरीरस्थेन देहिनाम्।
अव्यापन्ना: प्रसन्नेन रक्तमित्यभिधीयते।।
रसाद्रक्तं ततो मांसं मांसान्मेद: प्रजायते।
मेदसोऽस्थि ततो मज्जा मज्ज्ञ: शुक्रं तु जायते।। (सुश्रुतसंहिता-सूत्रस्थान 14.4-10)

49. भौमाप्याग्नेयवायव्या: पंचोष्माण: सनाभसा:।
पंचाहारगुणान्स्वान्स्वान्पार्थिवादीन्पचन्ति हि।।
यथास्वैरेव पुष्यन्ति देहे द्रव्यगुणा: पृथक्।
पार्थिवा: पार्थिवानेव शेषा: शेषांश्च कृत्स्नश:।। (चरकसंहिता-चिकित्सा 15.12-13)

50. रसनिमित्तमेव स्थौल्यं कार्श्यं च। तत्र श्लेष्मलाहारसेविनोऽध्ययनशीलस्य अव्यायामिनो दिवास्वप्नरतस्य च आम एव अन्नरसो मधुरतरश्च शरीरमनुक्रमन् अतिस्नेहान् मेदोजनयति, तदतिस्थौल्यमाष्मदयति।। (सुश्रुतसंहिता-सूत्रस्थान 15.38)

51. मेदोग्रन्थीन् शितै: शस्त्रै: पाटयित्वा समुद्धरेत्।
प्रवृद्धामश्मरीं शस्त्रै: पाटयित्वा नहि क्षिपेत्।। (1.19.288)

52. रक्तावशोधनं कार्यं नीरजाभिर्मुहुर्मुहु:।
तथा कार्यं प्रयत्नेन यथा पाको न जायते।। (1.19.198)

53. एरण्डश्च विदारी च वृश्चिकश्च पुनर्नवा।
स्नेहत्रयं पचेदेतैस्तल्लेपाद् विद्रधीं जयेत्।। (1.19.251)

54. एकमेवौषधं हन्ति दोषं कोष्ठसमाश्रितम्।
अपत्यं न गुणं किञ्चित् कुरुते तत् सुधासमम्।।
अजीर्यत्यौषधं यस्माज्ज्वरार्तस्य विनाऽग्निना।
तस्मात् दद्याद् भैषज्यं लङ्घनं तु प्रयोजयेत्।। (1.19.147-48)

55. M.Kripacharyulu Guntur, *Sāyana and Madhva* (Ph.D. Thesis, presented to the Karnatak University, Dharwad, 1977), p. 140.

56. ब्रह्मचर्येण तपसा निग्रहेणेन्द्रियस्य च।
जप्रेन ध्याना-मौनाभ्यां प्राणायामै: समाधिना।।
एतै: तपोभि: कुरुते नियत: कायशोषणम्।
स सर्वं लभते कामं दुष्प्रापं नात्र संशय:।। (1.17.123-124)

57. 'चरकसंहिता'-सूत्रस्थान 1.26-36.

58. 'चरकसंहिता'-सूत्रस्थाान 26.15-22.

59. तस्योपधातान्मूर्च्छायं भेदान्मरणमृच्छति।
यद्धि तत् स्पर्शविज्ञानं धारि तत्तत्र संश्रितम्।।
तत् परस्यौजसः स्थानं तत्र चैतन्यसंग्रहः।
हृदयं महदर्थश्च तस्मादुक्तं चिकित्सकैः।। ('सूत्रस्थान'-चरकसंहिता 30. 6-7)
60. *Bhagavad Gita*—17-8-10.
61. नेन्द्रियाणि न चैवार्थाः सुखदुःखस्य हेतवः।
हेतुस्तु सुखदुःखस्य योगो दृष्टश्चतुर्विधः।।
सन्तीन्द्रियाणि सन्त्यार्थः योगो न च न चास्ति रुक्।
न सुखं कारणं तस्माद्योग एवं चतुर्विधः।। ('चरकसंहिता' शरीरस्थान 130-131)
62. 'चरकसंहिता' सूत्रस्थान 26-10.
63. 'चरकसंहिता' सूत्रस्थान 26-12.
64. 'चरकसंहिता' सूत्रस्थान 1-51.
65. 'चरकसंहिता' सूत्रस्थान 26-43.
66. D.D. Mehta, *Positive Science in the Vedas* Arnold Heinmann Publishers, New Delhi, 1974, p. 86.
67. शतं ते राजन् भिषजः सहस्त्रमुर्वी गंभीरा तुमतिष्टेऽस्तु। (ऋग्वेद-1.29.9)
68. अधीतोरध्यगादयमधि जीवपुरा अगन्।
शतं हयस्य भिषजः सहस्त्रमुत वीरुथः।। (अथर्ववेद-2.9.3)
69. यत्रोषधीः समग्मत राजानः समिताविव।
विप्रः स उच्यते भिषक् रथोहामीवचातनः।। (ऋग्वेद-10.97.6)
70. प्रथमो दैव्यो भिषक्। (ऋग्वेद 2.33.3)
71. भिषक्तमं त्वा भिषजां श्रृणोभि। (ऋग्वेद 2.33.4)
72. रसायनक्रिया देषा कथिता पूर्वसूरिभिः।
कुटीप्रवेशनादेका वातातपसहा परा।। (2.1.14)
73. गोक्षरं बृहती द्वन्दा गुहा चातिगुहापि च।
एतैः प्रक्कथिता पेया श्वास-कास ज्वरार्तनुत्।। (1.19.162)
74. ऊर्ध्वं प्रवृत्ते रुचिरे पेया नैव प्रशस्यते।
ज्वरध्नेर्वा फलरसैः कृमिनाशं च वारुणम्।। (1.19.168)
75. भृष्टतण्डुलसिद्धापि पिप्पल्यामलकैर्युता।
यवागूः सधृता येषा विष्टब्धमलरेचनी।। (1.19.164)

4

ENVIRONMENT AND ĀYURVEDA

Right from Vedic times, though scholars have been thinking in their own way, it has not been possible to establish with certainty how the world was created or brought into being. This has been mentioned in *Nāsadīya Sūkta*. It is admitted as an axiom that the *pañcamahābhūtas* are the main cause or reason for the existence of the earth, and that these five elements control the world. The flora and fauna adjust the routines of their life according to the seasons. It is because of this that our ancients wanted the physicians to understand this phenomenon of nature. On the basis of this, they should conduct diagnosis. They should also understand how the earth was created, the role of *pañcamahābhūtas,* the *trīdoṣas* as also get acquainted with the general code of conduct. The environment these days is not being looked after properly by man. This has adversely been affecting the life of human-beings as also flora and fauna. Our sages never disturbed the cycle of nature and lived with nature. This enabled them to lead a healthy life of peace and plenty coupled with longevity.

Our ancestors believed in cosmic law. The relation between man and nature on the one hand, and the relation of cosmos with the ultimate on the other were well understood. The imbalance in any part of nature affects the life as a whole and, therefore, to maintain harmony among the members of the universe was felt a necessity.

Āyurveda as derived from compendia available at present, explicitly demands dynamic knowledge in environmental factors. The health, status and quality of life are directly related to status and capability of plant kingdom. When the plant kingdom is at the highest health status, the animals can enjoy health. The chances of availability of nutrition are based upon plants. By this communication, average intelligent person can choose or discard available materials for health depending upon status at that juncture. Even nutritiveness or non-nutritiveness of the materials was examinable by taste, and not by lab-gadgets. The multifactors of seasonal modifications provocate and annihilate certain things. So a health conscious person should know thoroughly the modification of seasonal stimuli and respond wisely to contact them. The entire health maintenance schedule is submission to mother Nature and never to turn as conqueror of Nature. The plant is to be prayed before it is taken for use. Individual possesses all the factors of the universe. Therefore, their preservation intact is obligatory for self-protection. Āyurveda, therefore, gives importance to eco-factors with reverence.

The environment is the sum total of all conditions with which man interacts in course of his existence. The total environment of man may be broadly divided into internal environment and external environment. The physical and the biological environment constitute the biosphere of the earth. Any area of nature where living substances interact to produce an exchange of materials between the living and the non-living environment, each influencing the properties of the other, are necessary for the maintenance of life.

There are two types of changes that are taking place in the external environment, changes in the structure of earth's surface and the changes in Nature of biosphere. Changes in eco-system, reshaping the topography of the earth, changing natural course of rivers, sinking of the earth and desertification are the main changes in the structure of earth's surface. Contamination of our water and land, accumulation of toxic wastes, destruction of forests and wild life, accumulation of carbondioxide and depletion of the protective ozone cover, are the main changes in biosphere.

Behavioural toxicology is a discipline that studies the harmful effects of chemical pollutants and pesticides, germicides, radioactivity etc. on human behaviour patterns and psychological well-being. It is obvious that so many chemicals in the environment pose problems associated with their measured or potential toxicity to both flora and the fauna of our globe. Environmental stress is a sub-branch of Environmental Psychology. Stress occurs in any situation when an individual perceives an external threat. Air pollution, noise pollution and hectic fast life are the causes of stress. According to Rājā Mānasollāsa mental stress is the main cause of ill-health. It is, therefore, necessary to lead a stressfree life by following a disciplined routine. This will help man to live in harmony with nature. Raja Mānasollāsa opines that the physician should curb his senses and dedicate himself to the service of *dharma* and well-being of his patient.

शस्त्रशास्त्रविदो वैद्यानभ्यास-निपुणानपि।
ऊहापोहविवेकज्ञान् सुधाहस्तान् प्रियंवदान्।।
अर्पयित्वा विचित्राणि भेषजानि पृथक् पृथक्।
निरालस्यांश्च धर्मज्ञान् प्रकल्प्य परिचारकान्।।

(2.19 139-140)

Man has eternally endeavoured to keep himself free from three types of miseries, namely, physical, mental and spiritual. Therefore, the history of medicine is as old as the history of mankind. According to Indian tradition, the four primary objectives of human life are : *dharma,* means to perform religious rites, *artha* means to acquire wealth, *kāma* means to satisfy the worldly desires and *mokṣa* means to attain salvation. Traditional systems of medicine developed in various parts of the world during different ages. A systematic shape was given to them in different ancient centres of civilization and culture. According to Caraka, Āyurveda or "the science of life", had always been in existence and there had always been people who understood it in their own way".[1] Some of these traditional systems are based on rational and sound fundamental principles and some others have only an empirical base. Some of those traditional systems did not survive and have become subjects of history of medicine like the Greek medicine and the Egyptian medicine. Some others, like the traditional systems of medicine of India and China, are not only surviving but also fully progressing.

Of the traditional systems of medicine in India, the practice of Āyurveda is prevalent in almost all parts of the country. Both in theory and practice, there are many things in common among these traditional systems of medicine of India. Each one of them has given to and taken from the other. The medicines of one system are, therefore, freely used by the practitioners of another system and these systems do not exist in water-tight compartments. However, Āyurveda is getting more popular among the people of India and it enjoys a unique position.

The word '*Āyurveda*' is composed of two Sanskrit terms, viz.,–'*āyus*' meaning 'life' and 'Veda' meaning the 'knowledge' and taken together, it means the "Science of Life" as has already been mentioned. However, in a limited sense, it is always used to imply "the Science of Medicine". Caraka has defined Āyurveda as the "Science through the help of which one can obtain knowledge about the useful and harmful types of life (*hita* and *ahita āyus*), happy and miserable types of life, things which are useful and harmful for such types of life, the span of life as well as the very nature of life".[2] It will be seen from this definition that Āyurveda lays emphasis not only upon leading a life of happiness, which implies an individualistic attitude but also leading a life which will be useful to society as a whole. Man is a social being. He cannot withdraw from society. Unless the society becomes happy, it will not be possible for the individual to attain or maintain his own happiness. It is with this in view that the individual should always make an effort to subscribe to the happiness of the society and Āyurveda texts are replete with references to the manner in which the society can be kept happy. The social medicine which is treated as a new concept in modern system of medicine, is nothing but reminiscent of what has been preached and propounded in Āyurveda more than 2500 years ago.

Āyurveda provides rational means for the treatment of many internal diseases which are considered to be obstinate and incurable in other systems of medicine in vogue now-a-days. Simultaneously, it lays a great deal of emphasis upon the maintenance of positive health of a normal or healthy person. It, thus, aims at both prevention and cure of diseases. For the purpose of preventing diseases, the regimens one should adopt during daytime, night-time and during different seasons, have been described in detail in Āyurveda. Man is exposed to diseases because of many external factors. But there are some diseases to which man is exposed even in the natural course of his living, e.g., hunger and thirst. Though they are basic needs of man, insatiable hunger and thirst may have to be treated as diseases. Āyurveda provides measures for the prevention and control of such extreme conditions.

Some scholars hold that *Pañcakarma cikitsā* (Five Elimination Therapies) is an additional branch of Āyurveda. Several classics were composed on each one of these branches and all of them were in practice. During the advent of Buddhism, practice of *ahiṁsā* became very popular. Surgical operations (which were invariably painful) were unfortunately treated as a form of *himsa* (injury) and thus the practice of surgery (*Śalya tantra*) was discouraged. This had an adverse effect on allied branches of medicine also. Thus, at present only three branches viz., *Kāya cikitsā* (Internal medicine), *Rasāyana tantra* (Geriatrics including Rejuvenation therapy) and *Vājīkaraṇa tantra* (Science of Aphrodisiacs) are in practice and the other branches of Āyurveda have become only subjects of history of medicine.

The physician must study the following basic principles of the Āyurveda system of medicine—

1. *Treatment of individual as a whole* : In modern medicine, more attention is paid to correct the afflicted part of the body. But in Āyurveda while treating a disease, the individual as a whole is taken into consideration. Not only the condition of other parts of his body but also the condition of his mind and soul are taken into account while treating the patient.

2. *Low cost of Medicine* : For the most part, Āyurveda medicines are prepared from natural resources which are available in the forests of the country. Therefore, these preparations are relatively less expensive.

3. *No foreign exchange involved* : Almost all Āyurvedic drugs which include herbs, vegetables, metals, minerals and animal products, are available in India. No foreign exchange is needed. There is no need either for foreign expertise or imported sophisticated equipments.

4. *Conducive to income generation* : In the past, physicians used to prepare their own medicines for treating of their patients. At present, physicians are having very little time to prepare their own medicines. Therefore, many pharmacies have been established in private and public sectors. But for establishing such pharmacies huge capital is not needed and most of the profit from such pharmacies goes to the workers who collect raw materials for manufacturing the medicines. It therefore provides means of livelihood to several people in general and poor people in particular.

5. *Free from toxicity* : Āyurveda medicines have centuries of traditional experience behind them. Therefore, they produce little toxicity in the human body. Even though certain toxic materials are used in preparing medicines, they are always

detoxicated and made more acceptable to the body before they are actually administered in the form of a medicine.

6. *Conducive to the customs of the people* : Along with medicines very often certain diet and regimens are prescribed to the patients. These diet and regimens are in keeping with the customs and traditions of the people. Therefore, they are not treated as alien.

7. *Psycho-somatic concept of disease* : Diseases are not considered as exclusively psychic or somatic. Psychic factors are always described as causes of somatic diseases and *vice versa.*

This has given rise to a psycho-somatic concept of all diseases in Āyurveda.

8. *Emphasis on Preventive Medicine* : Āyurveda lays considerable emphasis on the prevention of the diseases. Several Do's and Don'ts (पत्थ्य and अपत्थ्य) are prescribed for maintaining good health. Regimens for different parts of the day, night and different seasons for persons of different age groups and social status, are prescribed and described in greater details in Raja Mānasollāsa for the king as well as citizens.

The Rāja Mānasollāsa says, "आज्ञानरूपेण, या शक्तिः सर्वेषां मूर्धनि स्थिता।" (2.8.696). There is an unknown power. It controls the entire world. On this base, we think the universe as the wonderful creation by the mighty power described as God in various ancient works. About this universe, Lord Krishna says in the *Bhagavad-gītā,* "पितामहस्य जगतो माता धाता पितामहः।" (9-17)—"I am the sustainer and ruler of this universe, its father, mother and grand father." And he also says, "अहं सर्वस्य प्रभवो मत्तः सर्वं प्रवर्तते।" (10.8) "I am the source of all creation; everything in the world moves because of Me. It means—The whole universe springs from Him, exists in Him and disappears into Him and that He alone is its director and protector."

Creation of the Universe : Different philosophical thoughts of India are enshrined in the *darśanas.* These *darśanas* are divided into two groups. Those believing in the authority of the Vedas are known as *āstika darśanas* and those not believing are called *nāstika darśanas.* Buddha and Jaina schools of philosophy and the philosophy of the Cārvāks belong to the latter category. The following philosophical schools belong to the former category :

1. *Nyāya darśana of* Gautama
2. *Vaiśeṣika darśana* of Kaṇāda
3. *Sāṁkhya darśana* of Kapila
4. *Yoga darśana* of Patañjali
5. *Pūrva mimāṁsā* of Jaimini
6. *Uttara mimāṁsā* or *Vedānta darśana,* by Bādarāyaṇa

The collective name for all these schools is *ṣad darśana* (षड् दर्शन). All the ancient Indian sciences like medicine, astrology, astronomy, poetics and architecture are based on these *darśanas.* For explaining the physical and chemical activities, help of *Nyāya* and *Vaiśeṣika darśanas* have been taken in Āyurveda. To explain certain phenomena, the help of *Bauddha darśana* has also been taken. But to explain the process of creation of the universe and that of man, Āyurveda primarily takes the help of *Sāṁkhya darśana.* Of course, this has not been accepted *in toto* but with certain modifications.

According to Āyurveda, the universe originates from *Avyakta,* which includes both the *Puruṣa* (Conscious elements) and the *Prakṛti* (Primordial matter) of *Sāṁkhya darśana.* From this *Avyakta* the entire universe takes origin as detailed below :

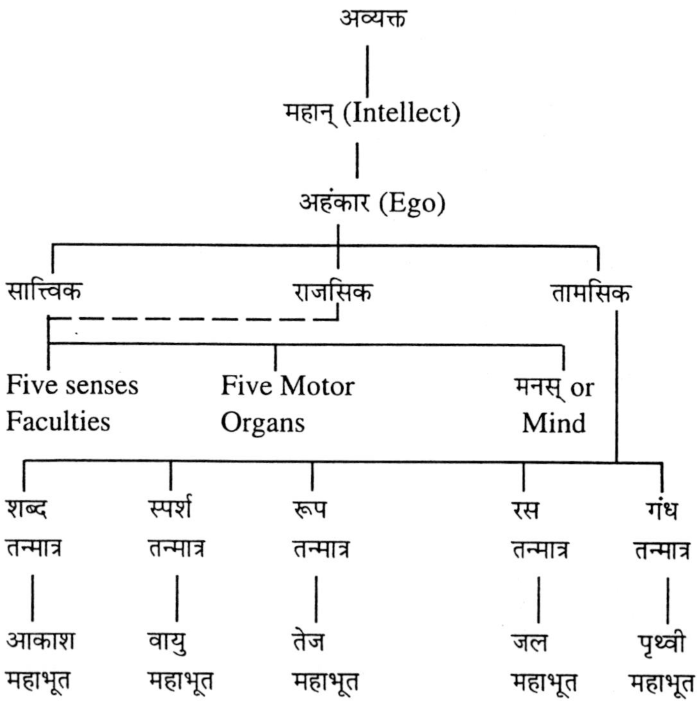

From *Avyakta* evolves the *Mahān* (Intellect) and *Ahaṁkāra* (Ego) follows it. Ego has three different aspects viz., *sātvika, rājasika* and *tāmasika. Sattva* is the purer aspect, *rajas* represents dynamism and *tamas* the potential destructive energy. *Sātvika* and *rājasika* types of *Ahaṁkāra* combine together to produce eleven *Indriyas.* The *tāmasika* and *rājasika* types of *ahaṁkāra* combine together to produce five *tanmātras.* From these *tanmātras* five *mahābhūtas* take their origin. From these five *mahābhūtas,* the entire material world—both animate and inanimate—is created. Inanimate world consists of these *mahābhūtas* alone and the living beings (including both plants and animals) are constituted of these *mahābhūtas* as well as *indriyas* which are eleven in number and include sensory faculties, motor-organs and the mind.

Pañca Mahābhūta are the basic cause for this Universe. Man has five senses and through these senses he perceives the external world in five different ways. The sense organs are the ears, the skin, the eyes, the tongue and the nose. Through these sense organs, the external object is not only perceived, but also absorbed into the human body in the form of energy. These five types of senses are the basis on which the entire universe is divided, grouped or classified in the different ways, known as the five *mahābhūtas*. They are named as *ākāśa* (ether), *vāyu* (air), *agni* (fire), *jala* (water) and *pṛthvī* (earth). The English equivalents given in parenthesis here do not connote five correct and full implications of these original Sanskrit terms. For example, ordinary water does not contain *jala-mahābhūta*. Similarly, air is not *vāyu mahābhūta* alone. It contains elements which belong to other *mahābhūtas* also. For example, oxygen will be nearer to *agni mahābhūta* and hydrogen nearer to *jala mahābhūta*.

Having described the evolution of matter from nature and its succeeding evolutes, we now proceed to the classification of the objects of creation in general. In this connection the *Sākhya Kārika* says.

अभिमानोऽहंकारस्तस्माद् द्विविधः प्रवर्तते सर्गः ।
ऐन्द्रिय एकादशकस्तन्मात्रपंचकश्चैव ।। 24
तन्मात्राण्यविशेषास्तेभ्यो भूतानि पंच पंचभ्यः ।
एते स्मृता विशेषाः शान्ता घोराश्च मूढाश्च ।। 38
सूक्ष्मा मातृपितृजाः सह प्रभूतैस्त्रिधा विशेषाः स्युः
सूक्ष्मास्तेषां नियता मातापितृजा निवर्तन्ते ।। 39
पूर्वोत्पन्नमसक्तं नियतं महदादि सूक्ष्मपर्यन्तम् ।
संसरति निरुपभोगं भावैरधिवासितं लिंगम् ।। 40
न विना भावैर्लिंग न विना लिंगेन भावनिर्वृत्तिः ।
लिंगाख्योभावाख्यस्तस्माद् द्विविधः प्रवर्तते सर्गः ।। 46

– (सांख्यकारिका, 24–46)

Self-apperception is egoism. From there proceeds only a

two-fold creation, viz., the eleven-fold set of sense and five-fold set of elementary rudiments.

The rudimentary principles are non-specific; from these five proceed the five gross elements, which are known as specific, since they are soothing, terrific and dulling.

The subtle body, which is primeval, unconfined, permanent and composed of intellect and the rest down to the elementary rudiments, migrates, enjoys not, and is not invested with affections.

If there were no conditions, there would be no subtle persons, and if there were no subtle persons, there would be no evolution of the conditions. Thence a two-fold creation proceeds, by name Personal and Objective.

These verses can be best illustrated with the help of the following table which shows all the stages in the evolution of creation.

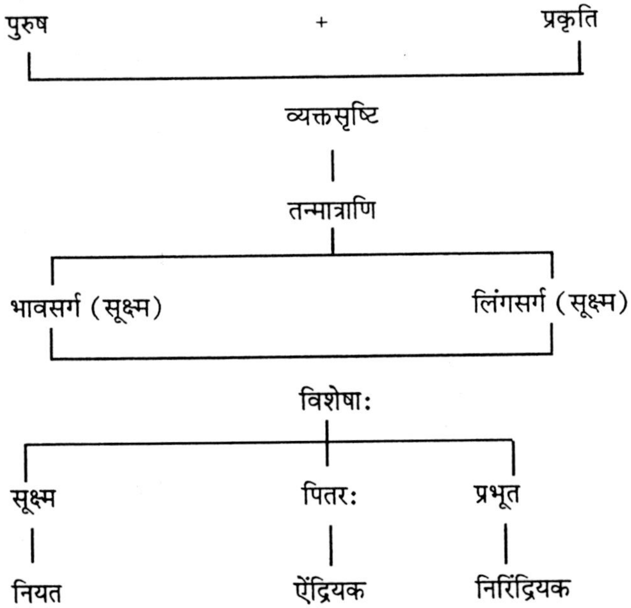

Classification of the Objects of Creation : Thus it will be seen that the *Sānkhya Kārikā* classifies bodies—substances—into two main divisions : (a) अविशेष (*Aviśeṣa*) Non-specific, and (b) विशेष (*Viśeṣa*) Specific. Caraka classifies them as (a) ऐन्द्रिय (*Aindriya*) and (b) निरिन्द्रिय (*Nirindriya*). We have to understand the *Aindriya* (चेतनद्रव्य) creation as consisting of combinations of subtle and gross bodies and the *Nirindriya* as (अचेतन), purely gross. The *Sānkhya Kārikā* classifies the specific bodies further into three divisions : (i) सूक्ष्म (*Sūkṣma*) subtle, and therefore everlasting, (ii) मातापितृज (Parent-born), and (iii) प्रभूत (*Prabhūta*)–diversified objects such as plants, stones, etc. The first of these, i.e., *Sūkṣma,* is rather difficult to understand and, therefore, needs amplification. The idea is that inasmuch as there are two facts, viz., (1) that the soul migrates, and (2) that the gross corporate body perishes, one has to presuppose that there is a non-corporal but spiritual frame which, being occupied by the soul, migrates from body to body carrying with it impressions (*Bhāva*) belonging to each previous life. Now we know that the soul being only a witness and a passive agent is not working actively with any personal interest. But this is explained thus :

It is always acting through the evolutes of nature and its reflections, such as *Buddhi* and *Ahaṁkāra.* As nothing, however, can proceed without a vehicular body carrying intellect (which again is subject to the influences of the *Triguṇas*) and as actions in life are followed by reactions in the next birth, we have to admit that there must be an intermediate rudimentary subtle body, लिंग-शरीर (*Lingaśarīra*), a receptacle or vehicle for receiving those impressions (*Bhāva*-भाव) and undergoing forms of life according to the respective *Karmas*. Both the rudimentary (लिंगाख्य) and the intellectual (भावाख्य) creations are attached to the same gross body till it perishes. The *Lingaśarīra* is the frame for carrying super-sensible set of Intellect, Self-consciousness, etc., but produces no intuition of it; the भावसर्ग (*Bhāva-sarga*) is the Objective Creation formed of conditions apprehended by means of senses, i.e., the assemblage of objects known by perception. Both these creations *(Linga* and *Bhāva)*, are not separable from each other but are interdependent, forming together the spiritual life. Thus, there is continual action and reaction going on between the states of Intellect and those of Body. Each conditions the other. As the rudiments premise the rudimental body, so the latter again premises the gross; for, we have already seen that without the gross body there can be no experience. It is because both kinds of bodies mean that the word 'विशेषैः' is used in *Kārika* No. 38 already quoted. In other words, Intellectual Creation cannot exist without a support and that support is the gross body bearing a corporal existence.

In short, the bodies, as we see in nature, according to the *Sānkhyakārikas* are specific substances containing both subtle and gross elements according to their requirement in the animate and inanimate creation. Modern science divides objects into 1. Organic and 2. Inorganic, which, in common parlance, are the same as animate and inanimate, respectively. Man, animals, vegetables come under Organic Creation. But only man is endowed with अध्यात्मगुणसंग्रह.[3] It is because of this unique quality in man he is able to lead a peaceful life free from strain and stress. Someśvara also highlights this quality in Rājā Mānasollāsa.

Modern physics and chemistry have divided matter into some basic elements. These elements differ from each other in certain points. All these elements can be classified into five categories of *mahābhūtas*. On the other hand, each atom has the characteristic features of all the five *mahābhūtas* in it. The electrons, protons, neutrons, etc., present inside the atom, represent *pṛthvī mahābhūta*. The force or cohesion, because of which they remain attracted towards each other, is the characteristic attribute of *jala mahābhūta*. The energy that is produced inside the atom when it is broken and the energy which remains latent in it in its unbroken form, represent the attributes of *agni mahābhūta*. The force of movement of the electrons represents the characteristic feature of *vāyu mahābhūta* and the space in which they move is the primary attribute of *ākāśa mahābhūta.*

According to Āyurveda, the body of the individual is composed of five *mahābhūtas.* In the human body, these five *mahābhūtas* are explained in terms of *doṣa, dhātu* and *mala* and in drugs they represent the *rasa* (taste), *guṇa* (qualities), *virya* (potency) and *vipāka* (the taste that arises after the digestion and metabolism of a substance).

In the normal body of a living being, these substances remain in a particular proportion. However, because of enzymatic action inside the human body, this ratio of five *mahābhūtas* or their equilibrium inside the body gets disturbed. The body has, however, a natural tendency to maintain equilibrium. It eliminates some of the *mahābhūtas* which are in excess and takes some of the *mahābhūtas* which are in shortage. This shortage of *mahābhūtas* is replenished through the ingredients of food, drinks, air, heat, sunlight, etc. The exogenous *pañca mahābhūtas* are converted into endogenous *pañca mahābhūtas* through the process of digestion and metabolism.

Even during the process of death these five *bhūtas* play a very important role. They have two different forms namely, gross and subtle. The five categories of subtle *bhūtas* inside the body impregnate the five senses for five times and thereafter, they get detached from these five senses and thus death occurs. The dead body loses the five senses and is composed, therefore, only of the five *mahābhūtas.*

Substances that are heavy, tough, hard, stable, non-slimy, dense, gross and abounding in the quality of smell are dominated by *pṛthvī;* they promote plumpness, compactness, heaviness and stability. Substances that are liquid, unctuous, cold, dull, soft, slimy and abounding in the qualities of taste are dominated by *jala;* they promote stickiness, like ointment, unctuousness, compactness, moistness, softness and happiness. Substances that are hot, sharp, subtle, light, unctuous, non-slimy and abounding in the qualities of vision are dominated by *tejas;* they promote combustion, metabolism, lustre, radiance and colour. Substances that are light, cold, unctuous, rough, non-slimy, subtle and abounding in the qualities of touch are dominated by *vāyu.* They promote roughness, aversion, movement, non-slimness and lightness. Substances that are soft, light, subtle, smooth and dominated by the qualities of sound are dominated by *ākāśa;* the promote softness, porosity and lightness.

In the organic world, these correspond to the *pañca-bhūtas* as and when operated by the soul. To be more explicit, the *pañca-bhūtas,* पृथिवी, अप्, तेजस्, वायु and आकाश, make up the whole of our physical matter, and this, when operated by the soul, is spoken of as being made up of *vāta, pitta* and *kapha,* which correspond respectively to *rajas, satva* and *tamas,* the *triguṇas,* which constitute the primal and fundamental triplicity of nautre—*prakṛti*—characterising manifested existence of all grades. The origin of *tridoṣas* from the five elementary substances is represented as follows :

तत्र वायोरात्मैवात्मा-------------------- वायुः

पित्तमाग्नेयम् -------------------- पित्तम्

श्लेष्मासौम्यः
अंभ:पृथिवीभ्यांश्लेष्मा] ---------------- कफः

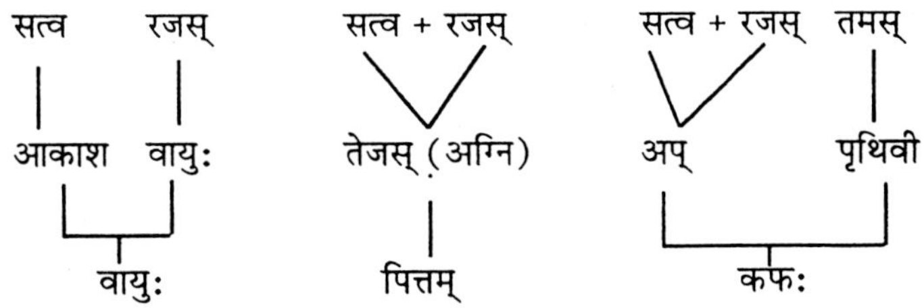

Suśruta describes the *tridoṣas* thus :

वातपित्तश्लेष्माण एव देहसंभवहेतवः। तैरेवाऽव्यापन्नेरधोमध्योर्ध्वसन्निविष्टैः शरीरमिदं धार्यतेऽगारमिवस्थूणाभिस्तिसूभिरतश्च त्रिस्थूणमाहुरेके। त एव च

व्यापन्नाः प्रलयहेतवः। तदेभिरेव शोणितचतुर्थैः संभवस्थितिप्रलयेष्वप्यविरहितं शरीरं भवति।।

-(सुश्रुतसंहिता-सू० 21-3)

It is from *vāta, pitta* and *kapha* that the human body takes its origin. They are respectively situated in the upper, middle and lower parts of the trunk and support the structure-body, just as three pillars support a building, and hence the name त्रिस्थूण given to it by some *Acāryas*. When they are diseased, they lead to destruction. So, with the aid of these three supplemented by blood as the fourth, the body is maintained in a normal condition.

Thus Suśruta gives here an idea of (1) what *tridoṣas* are, (2) what their normal function is, (3) how they take part in pathological processes, and (4) how with blood as a medium, they conduct all processes, from birth to death. He further observes—

विसर्गादानविक्षेपैः सोमसूर्यानिला यथा।
धारयन्ति जगद्देहं कफपित्तानिलास्तथा।।

(सुश्रुतसंहिता 21)

Here Suśruta compares the forces of nature with those of the human body. Just as the sun, the moon, and the air are heavenly forces in one sense and bodies in another, similarly, the *tridoṣas* which have गुण and कर्म are complex bodies having both anatomical and physiological functions in the economy of life. In other words, the *tridoṣas* are perfect *dravyas* and as such fulfil the requirements of *dravya* as defined by Caraka in यत्राश्रिताः कर्मगुणाः कारणं समवायि यत् तत् द्रव्यं। (चरकसंहिता सूत्रस्थान 1)

The substance, in which *guṇa* and *karma* are indissolubly united and which is a *samavāyi karaṇa*—समवायिकारण—combinative cause, is a *'dravya'*.

Now let us see what *dravyas* are. The history of evolution tells us that (1) the *tanmātras,* which are rudimentary principles and non-specific bodies, are *karaṇa-dravyas*—(भावरूप) करणद्रव्यs.

and (2) the specific bodies, which are the outcome-evolutes of the *tanmātras,* are *kāryadravyas,* कार्यद्रव्यs become organic or inorganic according as they are सेंद्रिय or निरिंद्रिय. All bodies, in this way, are naturally *Pañcabhautika* in their origin and constitution, but in the process of development where अग्नि is the chief working agent are marked off by changes in the qualities of the constituents. As the qualities changes, the results of the actions change.

The *dravyas* according to न्याय, वैशेषिक and आयुर्वेद are nine in number : 1. *pṛthivī*—पृथिवी, 2. *ap*—अप्, 3. *tejas*—तेजस्, 4. *vāyu*—वायु, 5. *ākāśa*—आकाश, 5. *kāla*—काल, 7. *dik*—दिक्, 8. *ātman*—आत्मन् and 9. *manas*—मनस्. Of these, the first five are, इंद्रियगोचर i.e., capable of being perceived by the senses, while the last four are not so, i.e., they are अतीन्द्रिय. All physical matter is *pañcabhautika* and composed of the five elementary *dravyas* mixed up in various proportions. The *paramāṇus*—परमाणुs of these *dravyas* are electrified particles belonging to these five elements, thus giving rise to the physical objects which we see around us. *Dravyas* are आकाशीय, वायव्य, आग्नेय, आप्य and पार्थिव.

At this point of discussion, it is to be noted that the *dravyas* do not by themselves explain the whole universe. They tentatively serve as their framework; it must be remembered that they are गुणवत्, कर्मवत् and समवायिकारणs. As compared with गुण and कर्म, they are नित्य. We have, therefore, now to consider the categories (*padārthas*—पदार्थs) other than *dravya.* By the term 'category' we have to understand, with the exception of one, the several groups or classes into which objects can be divided and not mere modes of predication. They are गुण—*guṇa,* कर्म—*karma,* सामान्य—*sāmānya,* विशेष—*viśeṣa,* समवाय—*samavāya,* and अभाव—*abhāva;* and together with *dravya,* they constitute the seven *padārthas* of the *Nyāya* school. Of these, *dravya, guṇa* and *karma* have real objective existence with them and therefore we are more concerned with them here. *Abhāva* is rejected by the Āyurvedists and Vaiśeṣikas.

The remaining are बुध्यपेक्ष, i.e., relative to understanding. We have already spoken about *dravya,* and we shall say a few words about each of the remaining six :

(a) ***Guṇa***[4] **:** *Guṇa* by itself is निश्चेष्ट i.e., inactive. It becomes a *Karaṇa* when it gets associated with *dravya* for the purpose of producing action. So, whenever we use the term *dravya,* we mean it, for all practical purposes, to be a combination of *dravya* and *guṇa.*

Guṇas are described by Caraka as "सार्था गुर्वादयो बुद्धिः प्रयत्नांताः परादयः". These belong to both *cetana*—चेतन and *acetana*—अचेतन *dravyas.*

अर्थाः	–	शब्द, स्पर्श, रूप, रस, गंध, Residing in पंचमहाभूतs
गुर्वादयः	–	गुरु-लघु; शीत-उष्ण; स्निग्ध-रूक्षः; मंद-तीक्ष्ण; स्थिर-चर; मृदु-कठिन; विशद-पिच्छल; श्लक्ष्ण-खर; सूक्ष्म-स्थूल; सांद्र-द्रव;
बुद्धिः	–	धीः, धृतिः, स्मृतिः, अहंकारः
प्रयत्नांतः	–	इच्छा, द्वेष, सुख, दुःख, प्रयत्न
परादयः	–	परापरतय युक्तिश्च संख्या संयोग एव च।

विभागश्च पृथक्त्वं च परिमाणमथापि च।
संस्कारोऽभ्यास इत्येते गुणा ज्ञेयाः परादयः।।

–(चरकसंहिता-सूत्रस्थान 26.27)

(b) ***Karma*** **:** *Karma* is defined by Caraka as

संयोगे च विभागे च कारणं द्रव्यमाश्रितम्।
कर्तव्यस्य क्रिया कर्म कर्म नान्यदपेक्षते।।

–(चरकसंहिता-सूत्रस्थान 1.52)

N.B.—Shows the general relation between the पंचभौतिकसूक्ष्मद्रव्य and the धातुs.

Prevailing तन्मात्रा	Prevailing type of द्रव्य	Prevailing दोष	Prevailing सप्तधातु in द्रव्यs	Physical & Chemical properties	Pharmacological properties	Physiological properties
गन्ध	पार्थिव	कफ	मांस	स्थूल,सांद्र, मंद, स्थिर, गुरु, कठिन.	मधुर mainly कषाय secondarily	स्थैर्यसंघातोपचयकरम् विशेषतः अधोगतिस्वभावं
रस	आप्य	कफ	रस, मेदस्, मज्जन्, शुक्र	शीत, स्तिमित, स्निग्ध मन्द, गुरु, सर, सांद्र, मृदु, पिच्छल.	मधुर mainly कषाय, आम्ल and लवण secondarily	स्नेहन-प्रल्हादन-क्लेदन बन्धन-विष्यन्दनकरम्
रूप	तैजस	पित्त	रक्त	उष्ण, तीक्ष्ण, सूक्ष्म, रूक्ष, खर, लघु, विशद.	कटुक mainly आम्ल, लवण secondarily	दहन-पचन-दारुण-तापन प्रकाशन-प्रभावर्णकरम्
स्पर्श	वायवीय	वायु	अस्थिन्	सूक्ष्म, रूक्ष, सर, शिशिर, लघु, विशद	कषाय mainly तिक्त secondarily	वैशद्यलाघवग्लपन विरूक्षणविचारणकरम्
शब्द	आकाशीय	वायु	आकाशीय commonl to al द्रव्यs	श्लक्ष्ण, सूक्ष्म, मृदु, व्यवायि, विविक्त.	अव्यक्तरस	मार्दवशोषिर्यलाघवकरम्

कर्म is a cause both in conjunction and disjunction, and it rests in a manner embodied in द्रव्य. Its function lies in doing that which is required of it to be done. It does not require any other condition.

In other words, कर्म is action pure and simple, and it manifests only when in combination with द्रव्य and गुण. Gangādhara, the commentator on *Caraka Saṁhitā*, says :

नहि निर्गुणं द्रव्यमस्ति न च अद्रव्यं कर्मास्ति।
ततः सहकारि कारणं द्रव्यकर्मणोरपि गुणः ।।

(चरकसंहिता-सूत्रस्थान 1-32)

Regarding कर्तव्यस्य क्रिया कर्म etc., he further says[5] :

"कर्म is independent of any other action alien to its purpose (स्वभिन्न) during conjunction and disjunction of स्वाश्रयद्रव्यs. It restricts itself to the same *dravyas*, brings about संयोग and विभाग by association and disassociation, changes the nature and properties of the *dravyas*, and eventually having undergone alteration, manifests itself in the form of an ordinary or extra-ordinary action, for the accomplishment of an act". *Karma* is both a कारणसामान्य and कार्यसामान्य, because संयोगादीन् हि जनयति कर्म। कर्म च संयोगोदिभ्यः जायते।

It must be remembered in the first place that *Āyurveda* is a practical science based upon realities in the working processes of the living human body. It cannot stand merely on abstract ideas. Therefore, Caraka, having stated in general the nature of द्रव्य, गुण, and कर्म, goes on to explain in the very next verse, what the line of action, i.e., medical treatment should be, as follows—

इत्युक्तं कारणं कार्यं धातुसाम्यमिहोच्यते।
धातुसाम्यं क्रिया चोक्ता तंत्रस्थास्यंप्रयोजनम् ।।

(चरकसंहिता-सूत्रस्थान 1-40)

He clearly states that द्रव्य, गुण and कर्म are कारणs and धातु साम्यक्रिया is their कार्य. He has already stated elsewhere that सामान्य

विशेष and समवाय are also कारणs. But considered from a physical point of view द्रव्य, गुण and कर्म are inseparable; some sort of गुण and some type of कर्म must accompany द्रव्य. On the other hand, सामान्य and विशेष are the causes of वृद्धि and ह्रास in द्रव्य; they change the गुण and कर्म in द्रव्य. So, द्रव्य is नित्य. in one sense, and गुण and कर्म (compared with द्रव्य) are अनित्य. All the द्रव्यs are not नित्य. They are of two kinds, viz., प्रकृतिद्रव्यs and कार्यद्रव्यs. The प्रकृतिद्रव्यs are the *Pañca-mahābhūtas* and the कार्यद्रव्यs are either सेंद्रिय or निरींद्रय. Instances of सेंद्रियद्रव्यs are शरीर, इंद्रिय and विषय. It is thus clear that the कार्यद्रव्यs are महाभूतविकारद्रव्यs, and not पंचमहाभूतs which are only original states of matter. Hence, we read the following words in Caraka "शरीरं नाम चेतनाधिष्ठानभूतं पंचभूतविकार समुदायात्मकम्।।"

Now समवाय indicates only a relationship between द्रव्य, गुण and कर्म. From a strictly logical point of view, it is a perpetual union, i.e., a condition of existence in which two things which are in a combined state, never had any separate existence. But समवायित्व changes with the कारणs, i.e., गुण and कर्म so far as the form and function of कार्य (शारीरिक) द्रव्यs are concerned. So. though समवाय by itself cannot be varying, the समवायिकारणs are varying. We thus, see the difference between पुरुष and प्रकृति, प्रकृति and विकृति, अविशेष and विशेष, सूक्ष्म and स्थूल and स्थूल and स्थूल. This view of the *Sānkhyakārika* corresponds with that of Āyurvedists and the Naiyāikas (नैयायिक). The soul varies according to the भावाख्य and लिंगाख्यसर्ग and constitutions vary according to त्रिगुणs (सांख्यकारिका). Following the same line of thought it can be said that त्रिदोषs are the products of पंचभौतिकद्रव्यs invested with qualities (गुण) and the power of action (कर्म). Thus, स्पंदन and उत्क्षेपण are कर्मs being the results of the action of वायु residing in the रजोगुण in a द्रव्य.

(c) सामान्य and विशेष.

(i) **सर्वदा सर्वभावानां सामान्यं वृद्धिकारणम्।**
ह्रासहेतुर्विशेषश्च प्रवृत्तिरुभयस्य तु।।

(ii) **सामान्यमेकत्वकरं विशेषस्तु पृथक्त्वकृत्।**
तुल्यार्थता हि सामान्यं विशेषस्तु विपर्ययः।।

(i) सामान्य, the common factor existing in *dravyas,* adds to their strength; but विशेष gives rise to a concept of their peculiarity consisting in separateness, as a factor leading to deterioration. Both these factors are simultaneously working, when in relation to the body economy. "प्रकृतिरुभयस्यतु" may be compared with प्रकृत्या च विरोधिना धातूनां वृद्धिह्रासौ भवतः। (च.शा.अ. 6)

(ii) "सामान्य brings about oneness or likeness, and विशेष difference, unlikeness or separateness. सामान्य indicates the fitness to accomplish a common object and विशेष indicates contrariety (अपचय)."

Gangādhara, the commentator, explains (i) सामान्य and (ii) विशेष in the following words :

(i) **समानानां द्रव्यगुणकर्मणां वृद्धौ**
प्रयोजकं सामान्यम्।

(ii) **विशिष्टानां द्रव्यगुणकर्मणां ह्रासे**
प्रयोजको विशेषः।

So. सामान्यम् वृद्धिकारणलक्षणम्, or एकत्वकरम् or तुल्यार्थता। (येन समानं यत् तस्य तेनसह तुल्यार्थत्वं-सामान्यम्)

विशेषः : असमानत्वं or विपरीतत्वं (अपचय) or
पृथक्त्वकृत् or ह्रासहेतुत्वम्

It must be noted here that the interpretation of सामान्य and विशेष in Āyurvedic literature is different from that adopted by the physicians of सामान्य and विशेष in the sense of genus and species.

In its highest degree (सामान्य), expresses only existence (सत्ता), a property common to all *bhāvas*. विशेष abides in the nine *dravyas* (पृथिव्यादि), which are eternal substances. Out of these nine *dravyas* आत्मा, मनस्, काल, दिक्, आकाश are infinite; and the परमाणुs of the remaining four, viz., पृथिवी, अप्, तेजस् and वायु are indivisible. They (अंत्यविशेषा:) have reached the uttermost point, and they are what they are by their indivisible nature. Its theory or doctrine is that all substances are composed of countless minute indivisible particles, from the combinations of which all forms of substances, physical and mental, arise, and from the operation of which all phenomena take place. These combinations are subject to change or destruction, but the indivisible particles cannot be destroyed or altered. This विशेष is the distinguishing feature of the वैशेषिक philosophy.

(e) *Samavāya* : Inseparable Inherence

In this connection Caraka says,[6] *Samavāya* is the perpetual intimate relation between an object and its qualities; in other words, it is the communion (fellowship) of two things, whereof one, so long as it exists, continues united with the other, e.g., this relation exists between पृथिवी and its गुणs.

(f) *Abhāva* : Negation or Non-existence

It is of four kinds :

1. प्रगभाव—Antecedent non-existence, as in the case of a pot before it is produced.

2. प्रध्वंसाभाव—Subsequent non-existence, as in the case of a pot after it is destroyed.

3. अन्योन्याभाव—Mutual non-existence, which finds expression in judgments like 'The pot is not cloth.'

4. अत्यंताभाव—Absolute non-existence; this variety we have when there is the bare ground with no pot on it.

In medical science *dravya* is to be understood as *Kāryadravya*, as it counts predominantly in the treatment of diseases. *Dravya* is, therefore, represented as *samavayikaraṇa*, i.e., combinative cause wherein actions *(karma)* and attributes (*guṇa*) exist. According to *Vaiśeṣikas* even soul (*puruṣa)* is a *dravya*, i.e., a substance, for, though it is devoid of action, i.e., change, still it appears to possess action by its contact with mind and the internal organs, in the state of phenomenal existence.

The human body, according to Āyurveda, is composed of three fundamental elements called *doṣas, dhātus* and *malas*. The *doṣas* govern the physico-chemical and physiological activities of the body, while *dhātus* enter into the formation of the basic structure of a body cell, thereby performing some specific actions. The *malas* are substances which are partly utilised in the body and partly excreted in a modified form after performing their physiological functions. These three elements are said to be in a dynamic equilibrium with each other for the maintenance of health. Any imbalance of their relative preponderance in the body results in disease and decay.

As has been stated before, inside the body, there are three *doṣas* which govern the physico-chemical and physiological activities. These three *doṣas* are *vāyu, pitta* and *kapha*. These *doṣas* are composed of *mahābhūtas*. All the *doṣas* have all the five *mahābhūtas* in their composition. However, the *vāyu doṣa* is dominated by *ākāśa mahābhūta* and *vāyu-mahābhūta*. In *pitta, agni-mahābhūta* is predominant, and *kapha* is primarily constituted of *jala* and *pṛthvī-mahābhūtas*.

The doctrine of the *doṣas* plays an important part in Āyurveda in as much as it forms the basis for the maintenance of positive health and diagnosis, as well as treatment of diseases. A correct appreciation of this doctrine is, therefore, essential for proper comprehension and appreciation of the theory and practice of Āyurveda. When they are in their normal state, they sustain the body and any disturbance in their equilibrium results in disease and decay.

These three *doṣas* pervade all over the body. There are, however, some elements or organs of the body in which they are primarily located. For example, the urinary bladder, the intestines, the pelvic region, the two thighs and the bones are the primary seats of *vāyu*. The seats of *pitta* are the sweat, the lymph, the blood and the stomach. Similarly, the seats of *kapha* are the thorax, the head, the neck, the joints, the upper portion of the stomach and the fat tissues of the body. Each of these three *doṣas* are again divided into five types. These five divisions represent only five different aspects of the same *doṣa* and they are not five different entities in the body.

Locations and functions of these divisions of *vāyu, pitta* and *kapha* are given below :

During different seasons of the year, these *doṣas* undergo certain changes. For example, *vāyu* gets aggravated during June-August, i.e., at the end of the summer. *Pitta* gets aggravated between October and December, i.e., during autumn, and *kapha* gets aggravated between February-April, i.e., during spring. If certain precautionary measures are not taken during these seasons, the person would expose himself to certain diseases caused by these *doṣas*. The precautions to be taken in these seasons will be described later. In the classical Āyurvedic texts, it is suggested that to promote positive health and prevent the occurrence of diseases, one should take medicated enema by the end of summer season, purgation during autumn and emesis during spring.

Factors Responsible for Aggravation of *Doṣas* : *Vāta* gets aggravated by the suppression of manifested natural urges : taking food before the previous meal is digested, remaining awake for long hours at night, speaking with a loud voice, physical exercise in excess of one's capacity, exposure to jerks because of travelling in a vehicle for a long time, intake of ingredients having pungent, bitter and astringent tastes, intake of dry fruit, excessive worry, sexual indulgence, fear, fasting, cold and grief. It also gets normally aggravated during the onset of rainy season.

Pitta gets aggravated by the excessive intake of pungent and sour things, alcoholic preparations, saline, hot, *vidāhi* (things which cause burning sensation) and sharp things. Other factors which are responsible for the aggravation of *pitta* are anger, excessive exposure to sun and fire, fear, fatigue, intake of dry vegetables and alkalies. Indigestion and irregularity in taking food also aggravates *pitta*. Pitta normally gets aggravated during autumn season.

Kapha becomes aggravated by sleep during the day time, by the intake of sweet things, cold things, meat, heavy, sour and slimy things, preparations of sesamum, sugarcane and milk, unctuous things, intake of food even after satisfaction, and intake of diet and drinks containing salt and water in excess during the spring season.

Aggravation of *vāyu* causes roughness, contraction, punching pain, colic pain, discolouration of the skin, malaise, abnormal movements in limbs, fracture, numbness, coldness, dryness and emaciation.

Aggravated *pitta* causes fatigue, sweating, burning sensation, colouration of the skin, foul smell, stickiness, anger, incoherent speech, fainting and giddiness. It is specially responsible for yellow colouration of the body.

Whiteness (paleness), coldness, heaviness, itching, unctuousness, *upadeha* (sticking of excreta in different orifices of the body), *stimitatva* (a subjective feeling as if covered with a wet cloth), *lepa* (a subjective feeling as if some extraneous material is adhering to the body), swelling excessive exudation and *cirakriya* (delay in action or response) are the manifestations of aggravated *kapha*.

Treatment of ailments caused by Aggravation of *Doṣas* : Drinks, diet, regimens and medicines which are unctuous, hot, stable, aphrodisiac, strength promoting, saline, sweet, sour, oils, exposure to sun, bath, massage, enema, inhalation therapy, sleep, taking rest, application of hot ointment etc., alleviate *vāta.*

Drinks, diet, regimens and medicines which are bitter, sweet and astringent, cold wind, shade, night, water, moon rays, underground residence, fountain, lotus, embracing the body of females, ghee, milk, purgation, sprinkling of water, blood letting, anointment, etc., alleviate *pitta.*

Drinks, diet, regimens and medicines which are rough, alkaline, astringent, bitter and pungent, exercise, spitting therapy, sexual indulgence, walking, fighting, remaining awake, aquatic games, *pādaghata* (putting pressure of different parts of the body through feet), exposure to heat and sun-rays, emetic therapy, fomentation, *upanāha* (application of hot ointments), etc., alleviate the aggravated *kapha.*

Environmental factors governing the upkeeping of a living body's capacity for resistance :

The environmental factors governing a living being are both external and internal. Air, water, place and time are external. Emotional imbalance and mal-adjustments are internal. The former causes physical disorders whereas the latter result in psychic aberrations. In normal circumstances, there may not be any cause for anxiety. In extra-ordinary circumstances, different reasons may cause different diseases. A shrewd physician, who knows both external and internal actions and reactions, exercises great caution in recognising and remedying the diseases.

The impact of air on the system is very important depending upon the season, e.g., in winter one experiences cold wind. In spring, it may be very slow. In rainy season it may be quite uncomfortable. At times, there may be gale or whirlwind with terrific speed or noise. When it blows carrying smoke or particles of dust, it is injurious for health.

Contamination of water is another factor. When water gets contaminated, it has foul smell with change in colour. Neither a living being bathes in it nor uses it for drinking purposes. Even animals living in water are affected by such water and suffer from diseases. Fish, tortoises, crocodiles, etc., suffer from it and grow thin. Even birds do not feel like tasting such water. Contaminated water causes ill-health.

A place or a country devoid of natural physical surroundings can be a source of health hazards and misery for living beings. A place full of reptiles, infested with mosquitoes, flies, rats, etc., becomes uninhabitable and such a place is unsafe for normal healthy being. Food grains may be destroyed. Unusual noise or sound of animals disturbs rest or sleep. Parched ponds and lakes, earthquakes and storms, piercing rays of the sun, change in the course of planets etc., are not signs of healthy surroundings.

Extreme climatic changes cause unusually hot or cold seasons, unusual rains or drought. These cause great misery for man, for animals, for birds and plants and herbs. In such a hostile surrounding, life becomes miserable and various types of diseases spread.

Science of life or Āyurveda suggests ways and means of combating such deadly diseases by proper diagnosis and effective treatment. By close observation, the sages in the past felt that change in air, water, place and time is inter-related. After analysis, a physician can determine how polluted air is the cause for water-contamination, how foul air and water make a place unhealthy and how such places affect the seasons also. It is through timely use of disinfectants, such pollutions are checkmated and impure elements eradicated.

For the purpose of eradication of diseases caused by various pollutions, a routine intake of diet, behaviour and movements have been recommended in Āyurveda. Prevention of diseases and promotion of health are the primary objects of this science of life. Cure of such diseases is also its another main objective. If a person reasonably follows the routine of diet, behaviour and movements, the cause of imbalance of *doṣa* is less. Diseases result only when there is mal-adjustment in *doṣa.*[7]

For maintenance of natural status of स्थान of *doṣas,* a routine for day—दिनचर्या, night—रात्रिचर्या and different seasons—ऋतुचर्या is prescribed.

दिनचर्या consists of rising early in the morning and meditating on one's chosen deity. After answering nature's call and doing physical exercise or performing *yogāsana,* one should have a enjoyable bath to eliminate the heat of the body and mind. After bath and worship of the deity according to one's faith, it is good to practise *prāṇayāma* to promote physical and mental well-being. Breakfast should be taken according to one's professional work, with devotion. After having nourishing and tasty fresh lunch, one should take some rest and again attend to one's legitimate work.

रात्रिचर्या consists of light work after evening exercise and taking dinner. Too many offsprings should be avoided to make the family small and contented. As the semen is the fine धातु and root of life, celibacy has to be observed for longevity and happiness. Sleep is known as भूवधात्री as it is the sustainer of creatures by removing the entire fatigue of the body and mind and restoring freshness.

रात्रौ किञ्चित् कार्यं कृत्वा भुक्त्वा च संविशेच्छ्यने।
नातिकठोर शुभ्रास्तरणे मशकप्ररोद्धियुते।
ऋतुकाले निजपत्न्या सन्तानार्थं व्यवायमथ कुर्यात्।
अतिसंन्ताने वर्ज्यः परिवारे सुखसमृद्ध्यर्थम्।।
शुक्रं चरमं धातुं जीवितमूलं नरः सदा रक्षेत्।
ब्रह्मचरन् खलु यत्नाद् दीर्घायुष्ट्वाय सौख्याय।।
निद्रा दिवसश्रान्तिं तनुमनसोर्हरति लीलयाऽशेषाम्।
येन पुनर्नूतनतां धत्तेऽतो भूतधात्री सा।।

(षोडशाङ्गहृदयम्–स्वास्थवृत्तम् 20–23 पृ० 253)

ऋतुचर्या comprises of routine for the six seasons. वर्षा—rainy season, शरत्—autumn, हेमन्त—early winter, शिशिर—late winter, वसंत—spring and ग्रीष्म—summer. The former three come under विसर्गकाल—releasing period while the latter belong to आदानकाल—receiving period. In the विसर्गकाल—releasing period, सोम—moon, is predominant. This promotes creation and strength. In the आदानकाल—receiving period, सूर्य—sun, is intense. He takes away all the sap or strength of living beings.[8]

ऋतुचर्या—seasonal routine, is very important. Various physiological symptoms of increase and decrease are visible in this period. So, each ऋतु, season, is described in detail so that both the physician and the patient may become aware of the possible changes and take necessary precautions before restoring normalcy or responding positively to the treatment given.

In वर्षा—rainy season, humidity is more, Digestion is slow. Due to faulty elimination of excreta, *doṣa*, वात, gets aggravated. In order to maintain digestive capacity, one is advised to take light diet. Old rice, intake of *ariṣṭas* mixed with honey is advised. Diet should be mainly of salts, fatty substances and sours which pacify वात. Drinking boiled or hot water is advised. One should avoid contact with contaminated water and also avoid sleep during day time.[9]

During शरत्—autumn, *pitta*—पित्त, accumulated during वर्षाऋतु gets aggravated. Piercing sun rays cause burning sensation resulting in पित्त disorder. So, sweets, bitters, cold and light items are necessary in the diet to pacify पित्त. Purgative is advised to eliminate पित्त. It is suggested to avoid sun-heat.[10]

During हेमन्त—early winter, digestive power becomes strong and able to assimilate even heavy items. There is no harm when one protects oneself against cold. Hot water bath after physical exercise is always good. Light diet, which aggravates वात, may be avoided.[11]

शिशिर—late winter, is the beginning of आदान—receiving period. The routine of हेमन्त is continued in this season with greater attention to protect oneself from cold and वात–

आदानकालप्रथमः शिशिरर्तुस्तेन रौक्ष्यप्रारंभः।
मेघप्रवातवर्षाजनितं शीतस्य भूयस्त्वम्।।

(षोडशाङ्गहृदयम्-शिशिरर्तुचर्या 43. पृ० 255)

In वसंत, spring, sun rays emit heat and so कफ accumulated in water gets aggravated.[12] Intake of diet consisting of wheat, barley and Bengal gram, physical exercise and hot water bath are advised.[13]

ग्रीष्म, summer, is a season when rays of the sun draw out the sap of living beings making them exhausted and weak. To counteract it, one should take rice with ghee and cold sweetened milk. Cold water bath is preferred and sleeping outside under the blue sky during nights would be pleasant. Sours, pungents, salty, hot, dry and rough items may be avoided in diet.[14]

The effect of air, water, space and time on a living body has been discussed in detail till now. Another important factor governing health is considered the trio of diet, sleep and celibacy. Just as आचार is परमोधर्म, आहार is परमो आधार of प्राण. Food is the source of life. Proper intake of food is necessary for nourishment. Strength, nutrition and contentment are the root cause of nourishment. Lest the body gets decayed by its self-destroying nature, nourishing diet becomes essential—

स्तम्भास्त्रयः प्रसिद्धा आहार-स्वप्न-शुक्रसंरक्षाः।
कायस्तिष्ठति तेषु प्रयतस्तस्मद् भवेत् पुरुषः।।
प्राणानामपि मूलं त्वन्नं पुरुषोऽस्ति नैव तेन विना।
अत आहारः कार्यो विधिना बलपुष्टितुष्टि करः।।
क्षणभङ्गुरं शरीरं प्रतिपलमपचीयते निजारब्धैः।
तत्पूर्त्यै बलशक्त्याधानार्थं ग्राह्य आहारः।।

(षोडशाङ्गहृदयम्-स्वास्थवृत्तम् 55–57 पृ० 256)

In an age when adulteration of food products is common,

it is very difficult to decide about a wholesome diet to nourish and replenish the decaying body. Although there cannot be a fool-proof nutritive diet, it is safer to follow the suggestions given in स्वास्थवृत्तम of षोडशाङ्गहृदयम्.

The Rājā Mānasollāsa gives detailed description of *dinacarya* (or time-table for the healthy person).

एतैस्तपोभिः कुरुते नियतः कायशोषणम्।
स सर्वं लभते कामं दुष्प्रापं नात्र संशयः।। (1.17.124)

It means there is no doubt that the person who does his duties regularly, with self-control, he/she should have healthy life.

One should get up from bed early morning. This is considered to be an auspicious time when there is less of noise in the atmosphere and the entire surrounding is impregnated with calmness and peace. Getting up from bed and offering prayer to the god (of one's own religion or belief) creates such an impact in the individual that he/she enjoys happiness throughout the day time. Before actually leaving the bed, an individual should chalk out his programme of work for the day.

Washing the face : Whether it is summer or rainy season or winter, one should wash the face with water immediately after getting up from the bed. This helps in the cleaning of the dirt accumulated in the eyes, nose and mouth during night and gives freshness. In winter season, lukewarm water can be used for this purpose.

Protecting Eyesight : While washing the face, one should take a mouthful of water, close the mouth and keep the eyes open as far as possible. A handful of water, with a little force, should be sprinkled over the eyes. This is considered to be very useful for preserving and promoting eye sight. Care should be taken not to apply much force while sprinkling water. After sprinkling water, eyelids should be very gently rubbed so that the eyeballs get a gentle massage.

Drinking Water : According to Rāja Mānasollāsa, the king should drink *divya* (rain) water in the *Śarad* season, flowing water from rivers in *Hemanta,* from lakes in *Sisira,* from big reservoirs in *Vasanta,* from springs *Vasanta* in the hot season and from wells in the rainy season.

दिव्यं शरदि पानीयं हेमन्ते सरिदुद्भवम्।
शिशिरे वारि ताडागं वसन्ते सारसं पयः।। (3-14.1627)

After washing the face and mouth, one should drink a glass of water. This is prescribed for all seasons and on all days. This helps in the proper evacuation of the bowels. Some people are in the habit of taking bed tea for this purpose. The reflex action produced by bed tea is different from the one produced by the cold water. Only the latter produces pressure, thus, stimulating the intestines to start the peristatic movement for evacuation. Tea (caffeine) stimulates the intestines so strongly that its stimulating effect loses its significance after some days and the individual becomes addicted to tea. The caffeine content of the tea or coffee produces some adverse effects on the glands of the stomach and intestines which the cold water does not. Cold water is, however, prohibited if the individual is suffering from cold, cough or sore throat.

Evacuation : One should make a regular habit of going to latrine after getting up from bed. One does not feel the urge for it at times, because of certain reasons. Either the meal of the previous night has not been properly digested, or the individual had inadequate sleep. The habit of drinking a glass of cold water in the morning overcomes these difficulties caused by indigestion and inadequate sleep and thus, the individual gets clear motion. People who are exposed to a lot of worry or those who are short-tempered, sensitive or wrathful, do get a lot of wind in their stomach. This accumulates in the intestines during the night. Wind is also formed because of the intake of pulses (*dāl)* and fried things in excess. Wind formation also takes place in persons who do not take leafy vegetables and fruits in adequate quantity. Whatever the cause may be, when the wind is formed it creates some obstruction in the bowel movement. The individual may at times feel that he has complete evacuation. But after some time, he gets the urge again and there are people who go to latrine three to four times in the morning itself, before they feel comfortable with the evacuation. This causes considerable inconvenience, and in many cases, the evacuation remains incomplete which causes suppression of appetite, indigestion, headache, uneasy feeling, fatigue and even sleeplessness. Wind, when formed in excess, puts pressure on the heart and may cause palpitation. It is, therefore, necessary for an individual to take necessary precautions relating to food, drinks and sleep, so that he gets clear motion in the morning. However, if he has an urge for the second time, it should not be stopped by force. That will not be good for health.

Cleaning teeth : One should use the tooth-cleaning stick whose top portion is crushed and which is either astringent, pungent or bitter in taste. This should be done in such a way that the gums are not injured. This removes the foul smell from the mouth. It removes the dirt of the tongue, teeth and mouth creating thereby the taste for food. In addition, teeth are kept clean and healthy.

Tongue scraping : Tongue scrapers should be made of gold, silver, copper, tin or brass. Their edges should not be sharp and they should be curved to facilitate scraping. The midrib of a mango leaf can also be used as a tongue scraper. The scum deposited on the tongue gives rise to foul smell. So the tongue should be scraped regularly.

Use of Nasal drops : One should inhale *Aṇu taila* every year during the three seasons, viz., the rainy season, the autumn and the spring, when the sky is free from clouds.

One who habitually resorts to nasal therapy in time according to the prescribed method, his eyes, nose and ears are not affected by any morbidity. His hair and beard never become white or grey; he never experiences hair fall; these rather grow luxuriously. Diseases like torticollis, headache, facial paralysis, lock jaw, rhinitis, hemicrania and tremors of the head are cured by inhalation therapy. Being nourished by inhalation, his veins, joints, ligaments and tendons of head and neck gain greater strength. His face becomes cheerful and plumpy and his voice becomes sweet and stabilised. All his sense organs become clear and they gain considerable strength. Diseases relating to head and neck do not attack him all of a sudden. Even though he might be growing old, old age does not affect his head in the form of grey hair.

Chewing : One desirous of clarity, taste and good smell of mouth should keep in mouth (chew) the fruits of *jāti (Myristica fragranas* Houtt.), *kataka (Hibiscus abelmoschus* Linn.), *pūga (Areca catechu* Linn.) *kakkola (Fiper cubeba* Linn.), *sūkṣmailā (Elettaria cardamomum* Maton.), flower stalk of *lavanga (Syzygium aromaticum* Merr. and L.M.), fresh betel leaf (*Piper betel* Linn.) and the extract of *karpūra (Cinnamomum camphora* Nees and Ebern.).

Application of oil : In this section, "the enjoyment of bath" and various kinds of preparation of an ointment are described. The king's personal attendants, Someśvara says[15], should first anoint the king with fragrant oil and then an expert wrestler, well-versed in the art of massaging, should massage his body. An ointment prepared with fragrant unguents like *koṣha* etc., in water or *kanjika* is to be applied afterwards to the body for rubbing and cleaning the skin. The scented oil of *āmalaki* should then be applied to the hair. Sometimes scented turmeric is applied in addition.

One who applies sesamum oil on his head regularly, does not suffer from headache, baldness, graying of hair, nor does his hair fall. Strength of his head and forehead is specially enhanced. His hair becomes black, long and deep-rooted. His sense organs work properly. The skin of his face becomes brightened.

Application of sesamum oil on the head produces sound sleep and happiness.

Oil Massage : As a pitcher, a dry skin or an axis of a cart, becomes strong and resistant by the application of oil, so by the massage by oil, the human body becomes strong and smooth-skinned. It does not become susceptible to the diseases due to *vāta* and it becomes resistant to exhaustions and exertions.

Vāyu dominates in the tactile sensory organ and this sensory organ is lodged in the skin. Massage is exceedingly beneficial to the skin. Therefore, one should practise oil massage regularly.

Of the person who practises oil massage regularly, the body, even if subjected to injuries or strenuous work, is not much injured. His physique becomes smooth, strong and charming. By applying the oil massage regularly, the onslaught of is aging slackened.

By massaging oil on the sole of the feet, roughness, immobility, dryness, fatigue and numbness are cured. It promotes strength and steadiness of feet. The eyesight becomes clear and vitiated *vāta* is relieved thereby.

Prevention of sciatica, cracking of feet, constriction of vessels and ligaments of feet are ensured if oil massage is applied to the feet regularly.

Unction over the body eliminates bad smell, curbs heaviness, drowsiness, itching and removes undesirable dirt and unpleasantness due to sweating.

Exercise : A physical action which is desirable and is capable of bringing about bodily stability and strength is known as physical exercise. This has to be practised in moderation depending upon the factors such as sex, age, climate, occupation, health, etc.

Good effects of exercise : Physical exercise brings about lightness, ability to work, stability, resistance to discomfort and allevation of *doṣas* (specially *kapha*). It stimulates the power of digestion.

Bad effects of exercise : Physical exercise in excess causes exertion, exhaustion, consumption, thirst, *raktapitta* (bleeding from different parts of the body), *pratamaka* (an acute form of dysphonia), cough, fever and vomiting.

Perspiration, enhanced respiration, lightness of the body, proper functioning of the heart and such other organs of the body are indicative of the exercise being performed correctly.

One should not do exercise, laughing, speaking, travelling on foot, sexual activities and night walking in excess, even if one is accustomed to these.

Contra-indication of exercise : Exercise is contra-indicated for persons who are emaciated due to excessive sexual activity, weight lifting and by travelling on foot and for those who are in the grip of anger, grief, fear, exhaustion and for the children, for the old persons and for persons having *vārika* constitution and profession of speaking too much. One should not do exercise while he is hungry and thirsty too.

Our ancient poets and scholars have given their appreciation on these topics[16] i.e., Physical Exercises :

1. Moving of mace or heavy weapons, bending bows, etc. provide exercise for the different parts of the body. This is known as exercise.[17]
2. Exercises, keeping the body fit, are considered the best.[18]
3. Enjoy wealth economically. Walk slowly and steadily. Climb up the hillocks slowly. Systematically cultivate learning and practise religion. Do exercise regularly.[19]
4. State revenue rises sharply when the king employs his energy within limits. Over-straining is the main cause of sharp fall. Exercises within the limits of bodily energy make room for sound health. Overdoing any thing results in dejection and loss of health.[20]
5. Oh! king, There is no other game which can equal

hunting. With a proper exercise, feet movement becomes quick and one can walk a long distance. It is very useful in times of danger for life. शीत (cold) is reduced and heat in the stomach, which is the main cause for bodily health, remains constant. With reduction of fat, physical organs become strong, fit and light. Resistance to cold, heat, air, rain, hunger, thirst develops.[21]

6. Posture is the first prerequisite in *Haṭhayoga.* Posture helps in steadying the mind and body, in maintaining health and in keeping them light.[22]
7. Person acquires honey through hard work. Hardwork alone helps him/her to get sweet *Udumbara* fruit. Look at the labour put in by the sun. He is ever moving without any exhaustion.[23]
8. One who sleeps, belongs to *Kaliyuga.* One who is free from sleep belongs to *Dwāparayuga.* One who is ever standing belongs to *Tretāyuga.* One who is ever on the move belongs to *Kritayuga.*[24]

Bathing : Rāja Mānasollāsa third *Vimsati* second *Adhyaya* explains about *snānavidhi.* Bathing is a purifying, sexual stimulant and refreshes the body and mind. It removes fatigue, sweating and dirt. It generates strength in the body and is an aid *par excellence* for the enhancement of the vitality in the body.

We find different views on bath in different works of Sanskrit literature. Some more information is given in the ancient Sanskrit literature[25] :

1. Neither cleanliness of body nor purity of mind-cleansing emotions—is possible without bath. So bathing is the prerequisite of physical and mental activities.[26]
2. Activities prescribed in Vedas, *Smṛtis* and Purāṇas are all religion-oriented and performed after bathing. So,

bathing is a daily requirement. It enhances charm, fitness and health.[27]

3. One should always take bath daily in a river, lake, tank, reservoir or a fountain.[28]
4. Fresh meat, fresh food, young lady, milk products, ghee and hot-water bath are considered instantly energising and inspiring.[29]
5. Morning bath, service of cow, gardening, working in flower garden and service rendered to parents are all considered sacred and healthy.[30]
6. Speak like a parrot. Meditate like a crane. Masticate like a goat. Bathe like an elephant.[31]
7. These are ten benefits accruing by daily bath : Strength, form, voice and colour become pure. Touch and smell become refined. Body becomes clean. Complexion improves. Youthfulness is retained. Beautiful brides are a certainty.[32]
8. Bathing keeps the mind cheerful, wards off bad dreams, strengthens the bases of sanctity, removes impurities, enhances lustre, beautifies form, wipes off an enemy, inspires warmth of love, helps in attracting women and relieves exhaustion.[33]
9. One should not take bath after taking food, while suffering from sickness, at midnight, putting on many clothes and in an unknown pool or pond.[34]
10. If sickness, weakness, old age etc. come in the way of bathing, do not pour water on the head. Either pour water all over the body or have a sponge bath.[35]
11. Implicit faith in one's religion is steadiness. Control of senses is religion. Removal of mind's impurities is bathing. Protection of the living creatures is charity. Bathing in water keeps the body clean. If it is not permissible, reading of holy texts, self-restraint and meditation can be practised to keep the mind tranquil.[36]

Dress : Raja Mānasollāsa explains about वस्त्रोपभोग: It says, excellent clothes of cotton or silk, woven with silver or golden threads of various kinds and colours, be brought from different countries and should be worn.

Wearing clean apparel adds to the bodily charm, reputation and longevity. It prevents inauspiciousness. It brings about pleasure, grace, competence to participate in conferences and good look.

Use of perfumes : Use of scents and garlands stimulates libido, produces good smell in the body and enhances longevity and charm. It gives corpulence and strength to the body. It is pleasing to the mind and it prevents inauspiciousness.

Use of ornaments : Wearing of gems and ornaments adds to the prosperity, auspiciousness, longevity and grace. It is pleasant and charming. It is also conducive to the vitality of the body.

The dressing and cutting of hair, beard (including moustaches) and nails, add to the corpulence, libido, longevity, cleanliness and beauty.

Use of footwear : Use of footwear is conducive to eyesight and feet. It protects the feet from attacks of reptiles, germs, etc. It gives strength and facilitates the display of physical force and is a libidinal stimulant. The author Someśvara deals with the interesting topic of *Pādukā Bhoga* or the enjoyment of sandals. After taking bath, the King should put on a pair of sandals made of *Śriparṇi* or *Harichandana* wood or of leather which covers only the front portion of the foot according to convenience. श्रीपर्णीदारुघटिते हरिचन्दननिर्मिते ।। (3.3.954-958)

Food : The Raja Mānasollāsa recommends change in food and drinks in accordance with the needs. One should eat in proper quantity. The quantity of food to be taken, again, depends upon the power of digestion including metabolism of the individual. The amount of food which, without disturbing the equilibrium of *dhātus* and *doṣas* of the body, gets digested as well as metabolised in proper time, is to be regarded as the proper quantity.

Items of food like *Sali (Oryza sativa* Linn.), *sāstika* (a variety of *Oryza sativa* Linn.), *mudga (Phaseolus mungo* Linn.), common quail, gray partridge, antelope, rabbit, wapiti, Indian sambar, etc.—even though light for digestion by nature, are to be taken according to the quantity prescribed. Similarly, preparations of flour, sugarcane and milk, *tila, (Sesamum indicum* Linn.), *masa (Phaseolus radiatus* Linn.) and meat of marshy and aquatic animals even though heavy for digestion by nature, are also required to be taken in proper quantity.

But from this, it should not be concluded that the description of heaviness or lightness does not carry any importance. The light food articles are predominant in the qualities of *vāyu* and *agni.* Those dominated by *pṛthvī* and *ap mahābhūtas* are heavy. According to their qualities, the light articles of food are stimulants of appetite and by nature are considered to be less harmful even if taken in excess of the prescribed quantity. On the other hand, heavy articles of food are suppressors of appetite and are exceedingly harmful if taken in excess unless there is a strong power of digestion and metabolism achieved by physical exercise. If the food articles are heavy, only three fourths or half of the stomach capacity is to be filled up. Even in the case of light food articles, excessive intake is not conducive to the maintenance of the power of digestion and metabolism.

Taken in appropriate quantity, food certainly helps the individual in bringing about strength, complexion, happiness and longevity without disturbing the equilibrium of *dhātus* and *doṣas* of the body.

Use of collyrium : One should regularly apply collyrium made of antimony because it is useful for the eyes. *Rasanjana* (a preparation of *Berberis aristata* DC.) is to be applied once in every five or eight nights for lachrymation of the eyes. Of all the *mahābhūtas, tejas* dominates in the composition of the eyes. So they are specially susceptible to the attacks of *kapha*. Therefore, the collyrium etc., which alleviate *kapha* are good for keeping the vision clear.

A strong collyrium must not be applied to the eyes during the day time as the eyes weakened by drainage will be adversely affected at the sight of the sun. Thus, the collyrium meant for drainage should, as a rule, be applied only during night.

Food is a must for all beings. But it should be proper and nutritious. Taittiriya Upaniṣad says, that[37] :

1. Food is the source of birth and growth. Anything swallowed by living beings is called food.[38]
2. Oh king! food helps in the birth and growth of living beings. All beings are alive by taking food.[39]
3. One can live long by giving up wealth which is not easy to renounce. But one cannot live long without taking food.[40]
4. Be upright in your action for procuring food. Take food only to sustain life. Protect life for continued existence of fundamental principles of philosophy. Cultivate dispassion and discrimination for wiping misery or sorrow.[41]
5. Consider food as creator himself. Don't condemn food. Follow this precept. Don't discard food. Follow this precept. Praise food. Follow this precept.[42]
6. The wise find no fault with food except when it is harmful to life or causes disease.[43]
7. Food deserves respect. It shall be taken without looking down upon it. Be happy and cheerful when food is served. Always speak highly of food.[44]
8. Food consumed is divided into three parts. The undigestible part is converted into filth. The middle

portion is reduced to flesh. The most delicate portion becomes the mind.[45]

9. Mind also becomes pure when food is pure.[46]
10. Of all cleanliness, clean food is the best.[47]
11. Water, food and wise-sayings are the three precious gems in this earth. But fools regard pieces of stone as gems.[48]

Code of General Ethics : Raja Mānasollāsa gives detailed description about ethics for Kings as well as common man. In addition to *Rājanīti,* these collections contain a primer of principles and morality of high ethical value many of which are generally accepted not only in India, but all over the world.

ऋतं वाच्यं प्रियं वाच्यं न वाच्यं हितमप्रियम्।
प्रियं न नानृतं वाच्यमेष धर्मः सनातनः।। (1.10.64)

One should not tell a lie nor should one take over others' properties nor should one long for other's wives or property.

अनायुष्यं परं नृणामगम्यागमनं स्मृतम्।
परलोके च भयदं तस्मात् तत् परिवर्जयेत्।। (1.3.44)

One should not indulge in hatred or sinful activities. One should not disclose others' defects and secrets. One should shun the company of the unvirtuous, traitors, lunatics, fallen persons, abortionists, mean and crooked persons.

One should not ride dangerous conveyances, sleep on a bed not well covered or without a pillow, small or uneven. One should not walk on the uneven slopes of the mountain, climb a tree and take bath in a river having turbulent flow. One should not tread on the shadow of kings or those born of noble families. One should not move around a place of fire, laugh loudly and release wind with sound. One should not indulge in yawning, sneezing or laughter without covering his mouth, itch the nostrils, grind the teeth, sound the nails, strike the bones, scrape the earth, cut the straw, grind the clod of mud and maintain improper position of different parts of the body.

One should not gaze at the planets or an undersirable, impure or condemned object. One should not transgress the shadow of a sacred tree, a teacher, a respectable person or an undesirable person. During nights, one should not enter the premises of a temple, a sacred tree, public courtyard, cross road, garden, cemetery and slaughter house. One should not similarly enter a solitary house or forest alone. One should not have relation with women, friends or servants of bad conduct. There should be no enmity with good men nor friendship with bad ones. One should have no choice for crooked acts. One should not indulge in ignoble or frightening acts nor should one take recourse to undue courage, sleeping, vigil, bath, drink or food in excess quantity. One should not sit for a long time with his knees up. One should not approach snakes or animals with dangerous teeth and horns. One should not provoke a quarrel.

One should not come to the fire without concentration of mind or without a wash after taking food. One should not heat his body by keeping fire below. One should not take bath unless he is free from exertion or in a naked condition. One should not touch his head with the apparel worn at the time of bath or strike at the tip of the hair. After taking bath, one should not wear the same cloth worn before. One should not go out without touching gems, feet of respectable persons, auspicious objects in left, nor keeping others in right side.

Study : One should not study if there is unseasonable lighting, while the quarters appear as if being burnt, during an outbreak of fire, earthquake, important festivals, fall of meterors, solar or lunar eclipses, on a new moon day and the dawn or dusk. One should not study without being initiated by a teacher. While studying, one should not recite words incomplete in sounds, in high voice, in hoarse voice, without proper accents, without proper morphological symmetry, too fast, too slow, with excessive delay and with too high or too low pitch.

General Conduct : One should not deviate from generally approved principles. One should not break any code of conduct.

असूयावर्जनं चैव पतितैः सङ्गवर्जनम्।
क्रोधस्य वर्जनं चैव स्वात्मस्तुति वर्जनम्।। (1.5.15)

One should not walk during the night nor in an inappropriate place. One should not indulge in taking food, studies, sexual relation or sleep during the dawn or dusk. One should not make friends with children, the old, the greedy, the fools, persons under afflictions or the eunuchs. One should not have any inclination towards wine, gambling or prostitutes.

One should not expose secret parts of the body. One should not insult anybody. One should not be conceited, undextrous, unfriendly nor should one indulge in backbite. One should not insult the Brāhmaṇas, nor one should beat the cows. One should not use harsh words towards the old persons, teachers, persons grouped together or king. One should not speak too much nor should one oust kinsfolk, persons attached, persons who had helped during the time of misery and those who know personal or family secrets.

One should not be impatient or overbold. One should not neglect the maintenance of servants. One should not have non-reliance on his own kinsmen. One should not enjoy alone. One should not have uncomfortable character, conduct, manners and diseases. One should neither rely on everybody nor suspect everybody. One should not be too meticulous at all times.

One should not be in the habit of postponing things nor should one indulge in any activity without proper examination. One should not be a slave to senses nor one should let loose his fickle mind. One should not inflict too much burden over the intellect or the senses. One should avoid over-dilatory practices. One should not do things in a fit of anger or rejoicing. One should not be under continued grief. One should not be conceited over achievement nor be desperate in loss. One should always remember one's own nature. One should have faith in the correlation of the cause and effect, that is, good and bad actions and their corresponding results, and should always act on it.

One should not be complacent about his own action. One should not lose spirit nor should one remember his insults.

Suitable Friends : One should have friendship with persons who have attained maturity by virtue of wisdom, learning, age, conduct, patience, memory and meditation. Those who are mature and learned, those who maintain the company of matured persons; those who are acquainted with the human nature, those who are devoid of all anxieties, those who are well behaved with everybody, those who are pacified, those who follow righteous course of action, those who advocate good conduct and those whose very name and sight are auspicious, are suitable for friendship.

नीतिज्ञं शौचसम्पन्नं व्यसनेष्वपराङ्मुखम्।
कुर्वीत नृपतिर्मित्रं धर्मार्थं सुखसिद्धये।। (2.7.686)

Unsuitable Persons for Friendship : One should shun the company of such persons who are of sinful conduct, speech and mind, backbiters, who are quarrelsome by nature, who indulge in sarcastic remarks about others, the greedy, who envy the prosperity of others, the cruel, who indulge in defaming others, the fickle minded, who serve the enemy, who are devoid of compassion and who do not follow the virtuous course of life.

Rātricarya : Sleep : When the mind gets exhausted or becomes inactive and the sensory as well as the motor organs are fatigued, the individual gets sleep. Sleep is nothing but the location of the mind in a place unconnected with sensory and motor organs. In the event of the exhaustion of the mind, the individual also gets exhausted because the actions of the individual are dependent upon that of the mind. Therefore, when the mind dissociates itself from its objects, the individual also dissociates himself from the objects of perception. As a result of this, the sensory and motor organs become inactive which leads to sleep.

Proper sleep endows the individual with happiness, nourishment, strength, virility, knowledge and longevity. On the other hand, improper sleep causes miseries, emaciation, weakness, sterility, ignorance and even early death. Untimely and excessive sleep as well as prolonged vigil take away both happiness and longevity.

Prohibition of sleep during daytime : Sleeping during the daytime in the seasons other than summer, is not advisable as it causes vitiation of *kapha* and *pitta.* Persons with excessive fat, addicted to taking unctuous substance, those with *slaismika* constitution, those suffering from *dusivisa* (artificial poisoning) should never sleep during daytime. If one violates the prescription regarding sleep during the daytime, he would subject himself to *halimaka* (serious type of jaundice), headache, timidness, heaviness of the body, malaise, loss of digestive power, *hṛdayogalepa* (a feeling as if phlegm is adhered to the heart), oedema, anorexia, nausea, rhinitis, hemicrania, urticaria, eruption, abscess, pruritus, drowsiness, coughing, diseases of the throat, impairment of the memory and intelligence, obstruction of the circulating channels of the body, fever, weakness of sensory and motor organs and enhancement of the toxic effects of artificial poisons. So one should keep in view the merits and demerits of sleep in various seasons and situations in order that it may bring happiness to him.

Indications of daytime sleep : Sleeping during the daytime in all seasons is prescribed for those who are exhausted by singing, study, alcoholic drinks, sexual acts, elimination therapy, carrying heavy weight, walking long distance; those suffering from phthisis, wasting, thirst, diarrhoea, colic pain, dysphonia, hiccup, insanity, those who are too old, too young, weak and emaciated; those injured by fall and assault; those exhausted by journey by a vehicle, vigil, anger, grief and fear, and those who are accustomed to day sleep. By this, the equilibrium of *dhātus* and strength are maintained and the *kapha* nourishes the organs and ensures longevity.

In summer season, nights become shorter and *vāta* gets aggravated in the body due to the absorption of fluid *(adana).*

Therefore, during this season, sleep during day time is prescribed for all.

The above-mentioned factors along with overwork, old age, diseases, specially those due to the vitiation of *vāta* like colic pain, etc., are known to cause sleeplessness even in normal individuals. Some are insomniac even by nature.

Measures to induce good sleep : If for some reason or the other, one is subjected to sleeplessness, he can be cured by massage, unction, bath, intake of soup of domestic, marshy and aquatic animals, *sali* rice with curd, milk, unctuous substance and alcohol, psychic pleasure, smell of scent and hearing of sounds of one's own taste, *samvahana* (kneading the body by hand), application of soothing ointment to the eyes, head and face, comfortable bed and home and in proper time.

Conduct during night meal : Food should be taken as early as possible during night. There should be sufficient gap between the time of intake of food and the time of going to bed. This will help in proper digestion of food which will result in good sleep also. The food should as far as possible, be light and easily digestible.

पथ्यं रुच्यं मनोहारि शुचि वृष्यं च भोजनम्।
माषचूर्णेन संक्लप्तं भक्ष्यं नानाविधं च यत्।। (5.20.1148)

क्षीरेण पाचितं पश्चत्सितया च समग्विनम्।
भक्ष्ययेत् सुन्दरं राजा भक्ष्यं भोज्यं मनोहरम्।। (5.20.1153)

Use of curds at night : Intake of curd during night is strictly prohibited. Curd is otherwise good for health. But it has a bad effect on the channels of circulation which are obstructed. This results in impairment of sleep and disturbance in metabolism. It is unsuitable specially for patients who are suffering from asthma, bronchitis and rheumatism.

Reading during night : With proper light, one can read books for sometime. But it should be clearly remembered that the artificial light of night is not at all harmonious with the requirements of the eyes. They ultimately affect the eyesight seriously. Thus, as far as possible, reading during night should be avoided or one should have light reading only. Writing during night seriously affects the eyesight.

Sex : Rāja Mānasollāsa states the qualifications of women whom a king should marry. Then it says, among the women, the beautiful one in full youth is the best and among the music-knowing, the dancer is the best. But at the same time, Someśvara says that it is difficult to get one with all the qualities mentioned.

One should not indulge in sexual intercourse with a woman during her menses or a woman who is suffering from a disease or is impure or is having infection or a woman with an ugly appearance or with bad conduct or manners or with the one devoid of skill.[49] One should not indulge in sexual intercourse with a woman who is not friendly or has not passionate desire or is passionately attached to somebody else or is married to somebody else or a woman of another caste. Sexual activity in any organ other than the genital organ is prohibited. Sexual activities are also prohibited under religious trees, in a public courtyard, on a crossroad, in a garden, at cemetery, at slaughter house, in water, in medical clinic or in the house of *Brāhmaṇas* or teachers or in temples.

Such activities are again to be avoided during the dawn and dusk and on inauspicious days (that is, on full moon day, *pratipada,* etc.). One should not indulge in such activities while impure or without having taken aphrodisiacs or without intense desire or without erection or without having taken food or with excessive intake of food or in an uneven place or while under the pressure of the urge for micturition, after exertion, after physical exercise, in fasts, having exhaustion and in places having no privacy.

One should make a habit to take a glass of milk added with sugar before and after sexual act.

Ṛtucaryā the two solstices : The year is divided into six seasons. The northward movement of sun and its act of dehydration brings about three seasons beginning from *śiśira* (late winter) to summer. The southward movement of sun and its act of hydration gives rise to the other three seasons beginning with the rainy season to *hemanta* (early winter).

The following table furnishes the details of various seasons :

Āyana	**Season**	**Months according to Indian Calender**	**Months according to English calendar**
Uttarāyaṇa (*ādāna kāla* or the period of dehydration)	1. *Śiśira* (late winter)	I Māgha II Phālguṇa	January-February February-March
	2. *Vasanta* (spring)	I Caitra II Vaiśākha	March-April April-May
	3. *Grīṣma* (Summer)	I Jyeṣṭha II Āṣāḍha	May-June June-July
Dakṣiṇāyaṇa (*visarga kāla* or the period of hydration)	1. *Varṣā* (Rainy season)	I Śrāvaṇa II Bhādrapada	July-August August-September
	2. *śarat* (Autumn)	I Āśvina II Kārtika	September-October October-November
	3. *Hemanta* (Early Winter)	I Mārgaśirṣa II Pauṣa	November-December December December-January

In the period of *visarga* or emission (hydration), winds are not very dry as they are during the period of *ādāna* or dehydration. The period of emission predominantly shares the qualities of the moon and during this period, the moon, with the unstrained cooling property, continuously delights the world with its soothing rays. The period of dehydration on the other hand, is dominated by the qualities of *agni* (fire). So, these three—the sun, the wind and the moon—being governed by time, nature and the path they follow—constitute the causes of time, seasons, taste in drugs and diet, vitiation of *doṣas* and bodily strength.

Effect of Ādāna Kāla on body : During the period of dehydration, not only the sun with his rays, but also winds with their sharp velocity and dryness, absorb the moisture from the earth. Winds progressively bring late winter, spring and summer, which enhance the bitter, astringent and pungent tastes respectively—all having drying effects and as a result, human beings also become weak.

Effect of Visarga Kāla on body : During the rainy season, autumn and winter, the sun moves towards the south, and his power of heating is slackened by various factors, viz., the time, course, storm and rain. The moon is, however, not affected. The earth is relieved of its heat by the rain water and drugs having sour, saline and sweet tastes, which cause unctuousness in the body, increase during the rainy season, autumn and winter respectively. As a result of all these, human beings also progressively grow in strength during the period of *visarga* or emission.

During the beginning of the period of emission and at the end of the period of dehydration, weakness prevails in human beings. In the middle of both, strength becomes moderate. However, at the end of the period of emission and beginning of the period of dehydration, human beings get considerable amount of strength.

Dietetics and Regimen for Winter : During the cold winter, the digestive power of human beings possessing good health and strength is enhanced due to the restraint caused upon it by the cold wind, so much so that it is capable of digesting any food stuff irrespective of its heaviness and the quantity. When it does not get the proper fuel, the digestive fire affects the nutritive fluids, resulting in the vitiation of *vāta* having cold quality. Therefore, during the winter, one should take unctuous, sour and saltish juices and the meat of the aquatic and marshy animals which are fatty. One should also eat the meat of burrow dwelling animals and *bhṛta* (a preparation of meat by mincing it) prepared of animals of *prasaha* type (who eat by snatching). Therefore, one should drink *madira*[50] and *sidhu* types of wine and honey.

If one habitually takes preparations of cow's milk, sugarcane juice, fat, oil, freshly harvested rice and hot water during the winter, his span of life is never decreases. In winter, one should resort to massage, unction, application of oil on the head and fomentation by *jentaka* process. One should reside in an underground residence or inside a heated apartment of the building.

In the winter, one should see that the conveyance, bedding and seat are well covered specially by heavy wrappers, skin, silken cloth, ropes and blankets. One should wear heavy and warm clothes and should besmear his body with *aguru* (*Aquilaria agallocha* Roxb.). One should embrace a healthy woman with her well developed and plumpy breasts, and with her body besmeared with *aguru* (*Aquilaria agallocha* Roxb.). Then he should lie down on the bed intoxicated with strong passion. One may indulge in excessive sexual intercourse during the winter. One should avoid food and drink which are light and which are likely to vitiate *vāta*. One should not expose himself to cold wave. Underfeeding and intake of gruel are also to be avoided.

The *hemanta* (beginning of winter) and *Śiśira* (late winter) season are almost similar in nature with the only difference that in the latter, dryness caused by *ādāna* (absorption) and cold caused by the cloud, wind and rains prevail. So the entire prescription for *hemanta* (beginning of winter) is to be followed in the *śiśira* (late winter) as well. One should stay in a windless and warm home—more so during the *śiśira*.

One should avoid taking such of the diet and drinks as are possessed of pungent, bitter and astringent tastes because they are light and they, therefore, vitiate *vāta*. During *śiśra*, one should avoid taking cold diet and drinks.

Dietetics and Regimen for spring : During the spring the accumulated *kapha* is liquefied by the heat of the sun and as such, it disturbs the power of digestion and causes many diseases. So, one should take therapies like emesis, etc., and should avoid heavy, unctuous, sour and sweet diet. One should not also sleep during day time. At the advent of spring, one should habitually resort to exercise and use unction and collyrium. The excretory orifices should be regularly washed with warm water. One should besmear his body with *Candana (Santalum album* Linn.) and *aguru (Aquilaria agallocha* Roxb.) and take food consisting of barley and wheat, meat of *sarabha* (wapiti), *sasa* (rabbit), *ena* (antelope), *lava* (common quail) and *kapinjala* (grey partridge).

Dietetics and Regimen for summer : During the summer, the sun evaporates the moisture of the earth by his rays. In that season, the intake of sweet, cold liquid and unctuous diet and drinks is prescribed. One who takes cold *mantha* (a type of groats) along with sugar as well as the meat of the animals or birds of arid climate, ghee and milk alongwith *sali* rice *(Oryza sativum* Linn.) during this season, does not suffer from any disease. One should either drink alcohol in a little quantity or should not drink at all, and even if one drinks, he should drink alongwith plenty of water. One should further avoid taking diets which are salty, sour, pungent or hot. Physical exercise is also to be given up during this season. During the night, after having besmeared the body with sandal paste, one should sleep on the open airy roof of the house which is cooled by the rays of the moon. One, decorated with pearls should be comfortably seated on a chair enjoying fans and the touch of tender hands—both cooled with sandal water. One should keep himself aloof of sexual intercourse and should enjoy gardens, cold water and flowers during this season.

Dietics and Regimen for rainy season : In the body, weakened during the period of dehydration the power of digestion is also weakened. It is further weakened due to the vitiation of *vāta* and other *doṣas* during the rains. The power of digestion in this period is also affected due to gas coming out of the earth, rainfall and increase of acidity in water. Consequently, *vāta* and other *doṣas* get vitiated. So it is advisable to be moderate as regards diet and regimen during the rainy season. One should abstain from taking *manthra* (groats) diluted in excess day sleep, frosts, water from river, excessive exercise, moving in the sun and indulgence in sexual intercourse. One should liberally use honey in preparing diet and drinks.

If the days are cooler due to heavy rains accompanied by storms, one should take such of the diet and drinks as are conspicuously sour, salty and unctuous. This serves as an effective antidote to the vitiation of *vāta* during the rainy season.

In order to maintain normal power of digestion, one should take old barley, wheat and *sali* rice (*Oryza sativum* Linn.), alongwith the meat of arid animals and vegetable soup. Moreover, one should drink the *madhvika* or *ariṣṭa* types of liquor, pure rain water or water from the well or pond, boiled and cooled, mixed with a little honey. It is advisable to rub the body, apply unction, take bath and wear fragrant garlands during the season. One should wear light and clean apparel and should reside in a house devoid of humidity.

आरोग्यमौषधाल्लभ्यमायुर्लभ्यं रसायनात्।
साहसाल्लभ्यते सिद्धिः कार्यसिद्धिरूपायतः ।। (5.19.976)

Dietetics and Regimen for autumn : The body parts adapted for rains and cold are suddenly exposed to the heat of the sun with the beginning of autumn. So, the *pitta* accumulated during the rains gets generally vitiated. In this season, sweet, light, cold and bitter food and drinks which have potentialities to alleviate *pitta* are to be taken in proper quantity when there is good appetite. Furthermore, the meats of *lava* (common quail), *kapinjala* (grey partridge), *ena* (antelope), *urabhra* (sheep), *sarabha* (wapiti) and *sasa* (rabbit), rice, barley and wheat are prescribed during this season. Intake of ghee prepared with bitter medicines, purgation and blood letting are also prescibed for this season.

One should avoid taking sun bath, fat, oil and meat of aquatic and marshy animals and alkaline, salt preparations and curds alongwith food. One should not sleep during day time and should not expose oneself to frost and easterly wind. The water is exposed to the heat of the sun during the day time and to the cooling rays of the moon during night. It is purified and decocciated by star Canopus (*Agastya*). This is known as *hamsodaka* which is spotlessly clear and is as beneficial as nectar for the purpose of bathing, drinking and swimming. Use of garlands made of autumnal flowers and clean apparel and also the rays of the moon in the evenings are exceedingly beneficial in this season.

Natural urges : The living body has some natural urges. They are the urge for (1) urination (2) defecation (3) sexual intercourse, (4) passing flatus, (5) vomiting, (6) sneezing, (7) eructation, (8) yawning, (9) hunger, (10) thirst, (11) tears, (12) sleep and (13) breathing caused by over exhaustion. They should not be suppressed. Inhibition of these natural urges leads to many complications which are required to be attended to properly.

Urge for Micturation : Suppression of the urge for micturation causes pain in bladder and phallus, dysuria, headache, bending of the body and distension of lower abdomen. To overcome these complications caused by the suppression of urination, one should resort to tub bath, massage, nasal drops of ghee and all the three types of enema (*basti)*.

Urge for Defecation : If one holds the urge for defecation, it causes colic pain, headache, retention of faeces and flatus, cramps in the calf-muscles and distention of abdomen. In such cases, fomentation, massage, tub bath, suppositories and enema should be given and one should take food and drinks which are laxative in nature.

The *rasāyana* or the rejuvenation therapies, prescribed in Āyurveda, are meant to remove these defects in the lives of old men. Caraka, while defining the scope of *rasāyana* therapy, has stated that the individual is endowed with longevity, memory, intellect, positive health, youth, excellent complexion, colour of the skin, voice, strength of the sensory and motor organs and lustre by its administration. In brief, the aim of this therapy is to maintain the youth of the individual along with his long life. Instead of a society of old and invalid people, it aims at creating a society of people with youthful vigour-both physical and mental.

Span of Life

The span of the life of an individual is divided into four parts. Upto the age of 20 the individual grows, the tissue cells multiply and the enzymes present in the tissue cells help in the synthesis of more tissues provided adequate nutrition and other congenial environment are provided. From 20th year upto the 40th year of life, the tissue cells continue to increase in number and quality. But this multiplication and growth is not so rapid as it was upto the age of 20 years. Man grows with experience. His field of activities increases, and thus, he is exposed to more strain and stress of life. He cannot be that carefree as he was upto 20th year of his age. The study period is going to be over. He is fully mature for marriage and for taking up a job. The creative faculty of his mind makes him worried to create new things and the ego in his subconscious mind wants him to surpass his colleagues and asssociates.

Marriage brings man additional responsibility of a life-partner, and the children thus procreated, are to be looked after carefully. He satisfies his biological urge for sex. The semen which is considered to be the most vital element in the human is lost. In Āyurveda a lot of emphasis has been laid upon the preservation of semen.

Celibacy or limited indulgence in sex is considered to be the *sine qua non* for the maintenance of good health of the individual. Whatever the ideal situation or concept of health may be, man is exposed to the vagaries of sex. The loss is well nigh replenished by the nurtrition he gets from his food. But this replenishment is always limited. The worry and anxiety to which man is exposed during this period of life starts affecting the functioning of the enzymes which are responsible for the synthesis of the tissue cells. He thus suffers. The physical growth is limited and is not in consonance with his mental activities.

From 40th year upto 60th year, is the age of stagnation. If the individual is provided with adequate nourishment, and if he is free from worries and anxieties in excess, he could maintain his health. The mental activities, no doubt, expand in dimension, the power of judgement increases and the sense of discrimination becomes sharp and acute. During this period, the individual should restrain himself from sex in excess, and if he does not do so, the process of decline of his physique starts even during this period. The process of ageing is manifested. The hair becomes grey, and at times, the head becomes bald. Wrinkles appear on the face and other parts of the body. One's capacity to indulge in sex becomes limited and the appetites goes down. Any vagaries in nature, like excessive heat, cold or exposure to rain, makes him sick.

The mental activities make him to spend sleepless nights. If he adheres to the prescribed conduct and resorts to wholesome regimen, he can lead a healthy life upto the age of 60. But there is no possibility of further growth of the tissue cells. Fat tissues may accumulate more and more, but this is not a sign of better metabolism. It rather indicates less power of the body enzymes to metabolise the nutritional food for the production of energy, and thus, they accumulate in abdomen, buttocks, neck and face.

From the age of 60 onwards, comes the period of decline. Whatever steps a person may take, the process of ageing cannot be prevented. His tissue metabolism goes down. More of waste products are found and inspite of best food, drinks and regimen, the body becomes thinner and thinner. His bones undergo change. Often there is osteporosis—lack of calcium in bones. The joints become dry and the fluid inside the synovial membrance between the two bone-ends gets dried up. The vital organs like heart, kidney and liver slow down their work. The nervous system becomes fragile and the arteries may be clogged. Thus, the man is exposed to ailments like high blood pressure, sleeplessness, enlargement of prostrate gland, rheumatism, cirrhosis of liver, osteo-arthritis, etc.

Any fracture of the bone does not heal quickly. He suffers from diabetes if the pancrceas slows down its work. The lens of the eyes become opaque and he suffers from cataract. The gums lose their strength and he loses his teeth. The nervous system stops working properly and he is unable to hear the sounds. His life beomes miserable and he becomes a burden on the members of his family as also on the society.

Our ancestors have given some suggestions, for good health,[51] as follows :

1. शीत (cold), उष्ण (heat) and वायु (breathing), these three are bodily elements both good and bad. When these are in unison or equal proportion in the body, such a body is called a healthy body. Equanimity, activity, and inaction form the three characteristics of the mind. A mind which constitutes these three characteristic in due proportion is called a healthy mind.[52]

2. A person, whose bodily functions as mind, heat and purgation are in harmony and whose soul, sense and mind are cheerful, is called a healthy person. Such a normal state is an indication of sound health.[53]

3. What is good fortune? Healthy mind and body. Who is truly a well to do man? An agriculturist. Whom does sin not trouble? One who meditates. Who is a complete man? A person with wise progeny.[54]

4. Fairmindedness, learning, health and satisfaction are

considered the best among virtues, wealth, benefit and happiness respectively.[55]

5. Oh! king, there are six types of happiness in this world—acquiring wealth, ever healthy body, loving wife with appealing speech, an obedient son and learning which helps earning money.[56]
6. Health, learning, company of the wise, birth in a reputed family and freedom from dependence are assets even without having money as commonly understood.[57]
7. An agriculturist is always free from want of food. A person with no disease is always happy. A householder with a loving wife is always full of gaiety.[58]
8. A healthy person does not want to go to a physician. Similarly, a king free from tension and danger, does not want to be in touch with a minister.[59]
9. Pārvati! Are you easily getting twigs and blades of *kuśa* grass for performing sacrifices? Is there facility for clean water for bathing etc.? Is meditation going on without any break? I am asking these because a healthy body alone is fit for religious practices.[60]
10. If a body is well guarded as a city, practice of yoga and attainment of bliss are automatically assured.[61]
11. Ignoring everything, one has to guard one's health—If health is lost everything is lost.[62]
12. Charity, religion, learning, physical charm, character, racial purity, health and fame, all these nine qualities have to be carefully guarded.[63]
13. Body is the foundation for maintaining health. At the same time, the body is the vehicle for contacting diseases. As the person directs the body to act, the body enjoys health or suffers.[64]

The *rasāyana* or rejuvenation therapy aims at keeping the enzymes in the tissue cells in their normal functioning condition. These cells are to be revitalised and their composition has to be changed. The tranquility of the mind has to be promoted and the nerves as well as bones are to be kept soft and soothened. This prevents the process of ageing and makes the individual free from any disease even during advanced age. He is able to see things as clearly as before and the sharpness of hearing continues. The glow in his face and the colour of his skin remains as before. It is with this in view one has to resort to rejuvenation therapy.

Time of Administration : Sooner the therapy is administered to the individual, the better. In more advanced age, this therapy just does not work well. Its effect becomes limited. Before starting the therapy, the following two points are to be observed :

1. The body of the individual is cleansed of the dirt or the metabolic waste products through specialised therapies, like purgation and vomiting.

2. He is taught to think, speak and work in such a way which would be conducive to the healthy development of the society. In fact, these conducts are given considerable importance in Āyurveda and they themselves are considered to have rejuvenating effects on the human body.

Method of Administration : This therapy is administered in two different ways. One is known as the *Kutipravesika* method while the other is known as the *Vatatāpika* method. For the former type, elaborate arrangements are to be made for the construction of a special type of cottage where the individual is to be confined. This type is, therefore, not suitable for a person who has to carry on his profession. For him, the latter type of rejuvenation therapy is indicated. He can resort to this therapy even while attending to his work.

Cyavanaprāśa : There are many pharmaceutical processes to make these drugs palatable and assimilable. The one commonly used by Āyurvedic physicians is *Cyavanaprāśa.* Āyurvedic physicians consider *Cyavanaprāśa* more a food than a medicine. All these factors depend upon the Nature. However, a physician must study ecology.

Ecology : Ecological imbalance is a debatable topic at present all over the world. Exploitation of natural resources in a callous or unsympathetic manner inspired by rapid advancement of technology, is the main cause for many environmental disorders causing misery to living beings. Felling of trees, building of high level dams across rivers, starting of small and large scale industries, inside as well as the neighbourhood of urban areas, are a few instances which are posing serious challenges to the survival of living beings. Forests are vanishing. Dams are causing quake shocks. Emission of filth into the rivers and pollution by smoke and chemical gases in the surrounding areas, are causing water pollution and atmospheric pollution. All this affects the health of the people inhabiting the localities around those complexes. These environmental disorders governing the upkeep of a living body's capacity for resistance have to be eradicated well in time to resotre normal health of the living beings.

Allergy is another factor causing grave risk for health of living beings. Perhaps even the medical profession is in the dark to find out the root cause of this allergy. Perhaps Āyurveda may provide a clue to this strange allergy through its accumulation and aggravation of *doṣas* and the remedies suggested for pacifying the same to restore normal health of human beings in the present day world.

It is not possible for anyone to live in an absolutely germ-free atmosphere. If the tissues of the body are strong enough to keep these germs at a safe distance the chances of their harming the human body are less. Granting that the body is affected by them, the tissues can be conditioned by diet and drugs to create a hostile atmosphere for these germs or bacteria not to survive, multiply or grow. Any accumulation or aggravation of वात, पित्त and कफ is said to be the main reason for bodily ailments. Rāja Mānasollāsa mentions a strange recipe for recognising these three, troubling the system. It is stated as follows—'Knowing the features of *Vāta, pitta* and *kapha* if pain is more it is called the effect of वात. If fever is more, it is called the effect of पित्त. If sloth or indolence is more, it is called the effect of कफ.'[65]

Intake of improper diet is considered as the cause of abnormal changes in the system. चरकसंहिता throws light on this topic—

न वेगान् धारयेद्धीमाञ्जातान् मूत्रपुरीषयोः।
न रेतसो न वातस्य न छर्द्याः क्षयथोर्न च।।
नोद्गरस्य न जृम्भाया न वेगान् क्षुत्पिपासयोः।
न बाष्पस्य न निद्राया निःश्वासस्य श्रमेण च।।
एतान् धारयतो जातान् वेगान् रोगा भवन्ति ये।
पृथक्पृथक्चिकित्सार्थं तान्मे निगदतः श्रुणु।।

(चरकसंहिता-सूत्रस्थान 7-3-5)

Someśvara says about लंघन-दोषकोपानुसारेण लङ्घनं विविधं स्मृतम्।। (1.19.153) In order to make the drug act positively, the science of life lays stress on अभक्ष्यवर्जन or पथ्यापथ्य in the cause of चिकित्सा. In order to facilitate the चिकित्सा or treatment, लंघन or diet control is advised. भक्ष्य, भोज्य, चोष्य लेह्य and पेय form the five components of लंघन. This is regarded as the preparatory stage of चिकित्सा in Āyurveda. Even the modern medical profession recognises the necessity of diet restriction. Food articles here are mainly classified according to chemical combination such as carbohydrates, proteins, fat, vitamins and minerals. In Āyurveda food items are classified as the basis of biological actions and their रस or taste.

Alongside bodily resistance, mental resistance also is of utmost importance to face the environmental factors. In fact, mental resistance is more powerful than physical resistance.

Mind controls the body. Intimate relationship of the mind and the body is a factor which can be ignored at peril. Physical disorders are normally caused by mental disturbances. Both require utmost attention in any type of treatment, be it native or foreign. Absence of mental worries always keeps the body fit to perform all activities. In Rāja Mānasollāsa the absence of mental worries is referred to by the term उत्साह.[66]

The concept of mind is considered very important to Āyurveda. It is also very significant in the system of योग. Body is regarded as the seat of disease in आयुर्वेद whereas mind is considered as the seat of disease in योग. Psychic factors always govern physiological functions of the body. Āyurveda has prescribed certain psychic treatment for controlling specific physical disorders. 'A healthy body and a sound mind' is an of repeated adage even today.

References

1. तदार्युर्वद यतीत्यायुर्वेदः (चरकसंहिता-सूत्रस्थान 30.23)
2. तत्रायुरुक्तं स्वलक्षणतो यथावदिहैवं पूर्वाध्याये च। (चरकसंहिता-सूत्रस्थान 30.24)
3. मनो मनोऽर्थो बुद्धिरात्मा च। (चरकसंहिता-सूत्रस्थान 8.3)
4. *Guṇa* is defined as समवायी तु निश्चेष्टः कारणं गुणः।। (चरकसंहिता-सूत्रस्थान 1-51)
5. सवाश्रयद्रव्याणां संयोगविभागेषु नान्यत्कर्मापेक्षते, तत्तद्रव्यमिवाश्रित्य संयोगविभागौ पुनः पुनः कृत्वा तानि द्रव्याणि तत्स्थांश्चगुणान् परिणमयत् स्वयं स्वयं च परिणमत् एकीभूय चिंत्याचिंत्य विशिष्ट कर्मरूपेण जायमानं समवैतीति कार्यस्य तत्कर्म।
(चरकसंहिता-सूत्रस्थान 1)
6. समवायोऽपृथग्भावो भूम्यादीनां गुणैर्मतः।
स नित्यो, यत्र हि द्रव्यं न तत्रानियतो गुणः।। (चरकसंहिता-सूत्रस्थान 1-49)
स नित्यो यत्रहि द्रव्यं = स समवायः नित्यः यत्र हि द्रव्यं नित्यम्
न तत्रानियतो गुणः = तत्र नित्येद्रव्ये गुणः न विनाशी।
7. आहारश्चाचारं चेष्टाः सेवेत मानुषो विधिना।
येन तनौ दोषाद्याः वैषम्यं नाप्नुयुः गदकृत्।। 4।।
(षोडशाङ्गहृदयम्-स्वास्थवृत्तम् Tr. Dr. P.V. Sharma p. 252)
8. वर्षाशरद्धिमान्ता ऋतवः शिशिरश्च माधवोग्रीष्मः।
पूर्वे त्रयो विसर्गस्तत्परे चादानकालः स्यात्।।

आद्ये सोमः प्रबलः क्रमशो भवति प्रवृष्टबलकारी।
अपरस्मिस्तु दिनेशः क्रमशः तैक्ष्ण्यात् बलं हरति।। *Ibid.*, 24-25 p. 253.

9. वर्षासु बाष्पदोषादग्निर्मान्द्यं भजेन्मलिनवपुषाम्।
दोषास्ततः प्रकोपं यान्ति विशेषात्तु गन्धवहः।। *Ibid.*, 26, p. 253.

10. वर्षासञ्चितपित्तं सहसा तिग्मांशुतीक्ष्णतरकिरणैः।
शरदि प्रकोपं गच्छत् दाहादिविकारकारि स्यात्।।
अन्नं पानं मधुरं तत्र विधेयं सतिक्तकं सुलघु।
शीतं पित्तप्रशमं मात्राकालादि सुविचार्य।।
पित्तस्य शोधनार्थं काले काले विरेचनं विधिना।
तिक्तौषधसंसिद्धं सर्पिश्चापि प्रयुञ्जीत। *Ibid.*, 33-35, p. 254.

11. हेमन्ते त्वतिशीते शीतमरुत्स्पर्शयोगसंरुद्धः।
अग्निर्भवति बलीयान् गुरुभोज्यद्रव्यपाक पटुः।। *Ibid.*, 37, p. 254.

12. शीतेनिचितःश्लेष्मादिनकरकिरणैः प्रकोपमुपयाति।
तस्माद् वसंतकाले कफजाः रोगाः प्रजायन्ते।। *Ibid.*, 45, p. 255.

13. कफशमनार्थं योज्यं भोज्यं गोधूमचणकयवयुक्तम्।
व्यायामश्च निषेव्यः शौचविधिः कोष्णसलिलेन।। *Ibid.*, 47, p. 255.

14. आदत्ते तु निदाघे सूर्यो निजरश्मिभिर्जगत्स्नेहम्।
अत एव याति कृशतां दौर्बल्यञ्चापि लोकोऽस्मिन्।। *Ibid.*, 49.
साम्लं कटूक्षालवणं भोज्यं ग्रीष्मे विवर्जयोन्नियतम्।
शुष्कं रुक्षञ्च बहु व्यायामञ्चातपे गमनम्।। *Ibid.* 54, p. 255.

15. औषधीगन्धसंस्द्धैः स्तुत्यैर्दोषापहैः शुभैः।
तैलैरभ्यज्य गात्राणि मलैः संताहवेदिभिः।। (3.2.933)

16. All these (1-8) statements are quoted from—Āyurvedāchārya Bhāskar Govind Ghāṇekar's "*Vaidyakīya Subhāṣita Sāhityam*", Chaukhamba Sanskrit Samsthana, Varanasi, 1977.

17. तुलभ्रमगुणाकर्षधनुराकर्षणादिभिः।
आयामो विविधोऽङ्गानां व्यायाम इति कीर्तितः।। (धनुर्वेद)

18. व्यायामः स्थैर्यकारणाम्।। (चरक)

19. शनैरर्थः, शनैः पन्थाः, शनैः पर्वतमारुहेत्।
शनैर्विद्या च धर्मश्च, व्यायामश्च शनैः शनैः।। (चाणक्यनीतिशास्त्र)

20. स्थाने शमवतां शक्त्या व्यायामे वृध्दिरङ्गिनाम्।
अयथाबलमारभ्भो निदानं क्षयसम्पदः।। (शिशुपालवध-2.94)

21. देव यथा मृगया ह्यौपकारिकी न तथान्यत् अत्र हि
व्यायामोत्कर्षादापत्सूपकर्ता दीर्घाध्वलङ्घनक्षमो जङ्घाजवः।
कफापचयादारोग्यमूलाशयाग्निदीप्तिः। मेदापकर्षादङ्गानां
स्थैर्यकार्कश्यलाघवादीनि। शीतोष्णवातवर्षक्षुत्पिपासासहत्वम्। (दशकुमारचरित)

22. हठस्य प्रथमाङ्गत्वादासनं पूर्वमुच्यते।

कुर्यात्तदासनं स्थैर्यमारोग्यं चाङ्गलाघवम्।। (हठयोगप्रदीपिका)

23. चरन् वै मधु विन्दति चरन् स्वादुमुदुम्बरम्।
सूर्यस्य पश्य श्रेमाणं यो न तन्द्रयते चरन्।। (ऐतरेयब्राह्मण)
24. कलिः शयानो भवति, संजिहानस्तु द्वापरः।
उत्तिष्ठंस्त्रेता भवति, कृतं सम्पद्यते चरन्।। चरैवेति।। (ऐतरेयब्राह्मण)
25. All these (1-11) statements are quoted from—Āyurvedāchārya Bhāskar Govind Ghāṇekar's *"Vaidyakīya Subhāṣita Sāhityam"*, Chaukhamba Sanskrit Samsthana, Varanasi,1977.
26. नैर्मल्यं भावशुद्धिश्च विना स्नानं न युज्यते।
तस्मात्कार्यविशुद्ध्यर्थं स्नानामादौ विधीयते।। (भविष्यपुराण)
27. स्नानमूलाः क्रियाः सर्वाः स्मृतिश्रुत्युदिता नृणाम्।
तस्मात् स्नानं निषेवेत श्रीपुष्ट्यारोग्यवर्धनम्।। (याज्ञवल्क्य)
28. नदीषु देवखातेषु तडागेषु सरःसु च।
स्नानं समाचरेन्नित्यं गर्तप्रस्रवणेषु च।। (मनुस्मृति 4.203)
29. सद्योमांसं नवान्नं च बाला स्त्री क्षीरभोजनम्।
घृतमुष्णोदकस्नानं सद्यः प्राणकराणि षट्।। (चाणक्यशतक)
30. प्रातःस्नानां, गवां सेवा आरामः, पुष्पवाटिका।
मातापित्रोश्च शुश्रूषा शास्त्राय च सुखाय च।। (महाभारत)
31. शुकवद् भाषणं कुर्याद्, बकवद् ध्यानमाचरेत्।
अजवच्चर्वणं कुर्याद्, गजवत्स्नानमाचरेत्।।
32. गुणा दश स्नानशीलं भजन्ते बलं रूपं स्वरवर्णप्रशुद्धिः।
स्पर्शश्च गन्धश्च विशुद्धता च श्रीः सौकुमार्यं प्रवराश्च नार्यः।। (महाभारत)
33. स्नानं नाम मनःप्रसादजननं दुःस्वप्नविध्वंसनं
शौचस्यायतनं मलापहरणं संवर्धनं तेजसः।
रूपद्योतकरं रिपुप्रमथनं कामाग्निसंदीपनं
नारीणां च मनोहरं श्रमहरं स्नाने दशैते गुणाः। (चाणक्यराजनीति)
34. न स्नानमाचरेद् भुक्त्वा नातुरो न महानिशि।
न वासोभिः सहाजस्रं, नाविज्ञाते जलाशये।। (मनुस्मृति 4.129)
35. अशिरस्कं भवेत् स्नानं स्नानाशक्तौ तु कर्मिणाम्।
आर्द्रेण वाससा वा स्यान्मार्जनं दैहिकं विदुः।। (जाबालस्मृतिः)
36. स्वधर्मे स्थिरता स्थैर्यं, धर्ममिन्द्रियनिग्रहः।
स्नानं मनोमलत्यागो, दानं वै भूतरक्षणम्।।
न जलाप्लुतदेहस्य स्नानमित्यभिधीयते।
स स्नातो यो दमस्नातः शुचिशुद्धमनोमलः।। (महाभारत)
37. All these (1-11) statemenets are quoted from—Āyurvedāchārya Bhāskar Govind Ghāṇekar's *"Vaidyakīya Subhāṣita Sāhityam"*, Chaukhamba Sanskrit Samsthana, Varanasi,1977.

38. अन्नाद् भूतानि जायन्ते; जातान्यन्नेन वर्धन्ते।
अद्यतेऽत्ति च भूतानि; तस्मादन्नं तदुच्यते।।
(तैत्तिरीयोपनिषद् ब्राह्मानन्दवल्ली -अनुवाक् 2.1)
39. आहारात्सर्वभूतानि सम्भवन्ति महीपते।
आहारेण विवर्धन्ते तेन जीवन्ति जन्तवः।। (महाभारत)
40. शक्यते दूस्त्यजेऽप्यर्थे चिररात्राय जीवितुम्।
न तु भोजनमुत्सृज्य शक्यं वर्तयितुं चिरम्।। (महाभारत)
41. अन्नाहारार्थं कर्म कुर्यादनिन्द्यं कुर्यादाहारं प्राणसन्धारणार्थम्।
प्राणाः सन्धार्यास्तत्त्वजिज्ञासनार्थं तत्त्वं जिज्ञास्यं येन भूयो न दुःखम्।। (योगवाशिष्ठ)
42. अन्नं ब्रह्मेति व्यजानात्।। अन्नं न निन्द्यात्।।
अन्नं न परिचक्षीत, तद्व्रतम्।। अन्नं बहु कुर्वीत, तद्व्रतम्।
(तैत्तिरीयोपनिषद् ब्रह्मानन्दवल्ली-अनुवाक 2.1)
43. उपघातमृते दोषं नान्नस्योदीरयेद्बुधः।। (मार्कण्डेयपुराण)
44. पूजयेदशनं नित्यमद्याच्चैतदकुत्सयन्।
दृष्ट्वा हृष्येत् प्रसीदेच्च प्रतिनन्देच्च सर्वशः।। (मनुस्मृति 2.54)
45. अन्नमशितं त्रेता विधीयते, तस्य यः स्थविष्ठो धातुस्तत्पुरीषं
भवति, यो मध्यमस्तन्माःसं, योऽणिष्ठस्तन्मनः।। (छान्दोग्योपनिषद्)
46. आहारशुद्धौ सत्त्वशुद्धिः। (छान्दोग्योपनिषद्)
47. सर्वेषामेव शौचनामन्नशौचं विशिष्यते। (बृहस्पति)
48. पृथिव्यां त्रीणि रत्नानि जलमन्नं सुभाषितम्।
मूढैः पाषाणखण्डेषु रत्नसंज्ञा विधीयते।। (वृद्धचाणक्य)
49. पुष्पिता पतिता कन्या लिङ्गिता श्रेष्ठजातिजा।
परस्त्री विधवा श्वश्रूः स्वसा त दुहिता तथा।। (1.3.42)
50. सुरसा जायते तेन सा मनोत्वकारिणि
क्षुधिते भोजनं मिष्टं तोयपानं तृषातुरे।
निदाधे शीतलं रुच्यं शीते धर्मः सुखावहः
इति मत्वा महीपालो यतेत प्रेमवर्धने।। (5.19.1025)
51. All these (1-13) statements are quoted from—Āyurvedāchārya Bhāskar Govind Ghāṇekar's "*Vaidakīya Subhāṣita Sāhityam*", Chaukhamba Sanskrit Samsthana, Varanasi, 1977.
52. शीतोष्णे चैव वायुश्च त्रयः शारीरजा गुणाः।
तेषां गुणानां साम्यं यत्तदाहुः स्वास्थ्यलक्षणम्।।
सत्त्वं रजस्तम इति मानसाः स्युस्त्रयो गुणाः।
तेषां गुणानां साम्य यत्तदाहुः स्वास्थ्यलक्षणम्।। (महाभारत)
53. समदोशः समाग्निश्च समधातुमलक्रियः।
प्रसन्नात्मेन्द्रियमनाः स्वस्थ इत्यभिधीयते।। (सुश्रुत)

54. किं भाग्यं देहवतामारोग्यं क: फली कृषिकृत्।
कस्य न पापं? जपत: क: पूर्णो? य: प्रजावान् स्यात्।। (शंकराचार्य कृतं स्तोत्रम्)

55. धन्यानामुत्तमं दाक्ष्यं, धनानामुत्तमं श्रुतम्।
लाभानां श्रेष्ठमारोग्यं सुखानां तुष्टिरुत्तमा।। (महाभारत)

56. अर्थागमो नित्यमरोगिता च।
प्रिया च भार्या प्रियवादिनी च।।
वश्यश्च पुत्रोऽर्थकरी च विद्या
षड् जीवलोकस्य सुखानि राजन्।। (महाभारत)

57. आरोग्यं विद्वता सज्जनमैत्री महाकुल जन्म।
स्वाधीनता च पुंसां महदैश्वर्यं विनाप्यर्थैः।। (शार्ङ्गधरपद्धति:)

58. सुभिक्षं कृषके नित्यं, नित्यं सुखमरोगिणि।
भार्या भर्तु: प्रिया यस्य तस्य नित्योत्सवं गृहम्।। (चाणक्यशतकम्)

59. यथा नेच्छति नीरोग: कदाचित् सुचिकित्सकम्।
तथाऽऽपद्रहितो राजा सचिवं नाभिवाञ्छति।। (पञ्चतन्त्रम्)

60. अपि क्रियार्थं सुलभं समित्कुशं
जलान्यपि स्नानविधिक्षमाणि ते।।

अपि स्वशक्त्या तपसि प्रवर्तसे
शरीरमाद्यं खलु धर्मसाधनम्।। (कुमारसम्भवम्)

61. पुरस्य दाढर्ये योगस्य सिद्धि: सर्वार्थसाधनी।
अखण्डानन्दसिद्धिश्च फलं तेनैव जायते।। (जीवानन्द)

62. सर्वमेव परित्यज्य शरीरमनुपालयेत्।
शरीरस्य प्रणष्टस्य सर्वमेव विनश्यति।। (चाणक्यराजनीतिशास्त्रम्)

63. दानं धर्मश्च विद्या च रूपं शीलं कुलं तथा।
सुखमायुर्यशश्चैव नव गोप्यानि यत्नत:।। (चाणक्यनीतिशास्त्रम्)

64. शरीरमेवायतनं सुखस्य दु:खस्य चाप्यायतनं शरीरम्।
यद्यच्छरीरेण करोति कर्म तैनेव देही समुपाश्नुते तत्।। (सुभाषितावलि)

65. वात-पित्त-बलासानां ज्ञात्वा लक्षणमुत्कटम्।
तस्योपशमनैर्द्रव्यै: कृत्वा पेयं प्रदापयेत्।।
वात: शूलेऽधिके ज्ञेयस्तापे पित्तं च लक्षयेत्।
जाड्ये कफं विजानीयान्मिश्रे मिश्रं तु लक्षयेत्।। (1.19.157-158)

66. प्रारब्धं यत् स्वयं कार्यं दैवाद् यदि न सिध्यति।
न सीदति च तत्कर्तुमुत्साही च पुन: पुन:।।
यस्य स्यादुद्यमे नित्यं चित्तमुत्साहसंयुतम्।
उत्साहशक्ति: सा ज्ञेया नृपाणां भूतिमिच्छताम्।। (2.10.723-724)

5

SIGNIFICANCE OF PHYSICAL AND MENTAL HEALTH

(According to Rāja Mānasollāsa)

"Prevention is better than cure" is a famous saying. Science of life—आयुर्वेद—goes a step further and makes both prevention and cure as its twin objectives. Prevention of diseases is necessary for promotion of health. When attempts to prevent diseases do not yield the desired result, methods to cure become necessary for restoring normal status in the system. Proper diagnosis and selective drugs are no doubt very helpful in this curative process. The role of diet is no less helpful and beneficial in the case of a patient for whom such drugs are prescribed. Drugs prove counter productive without the intake of nourishing and timely diet. Therefore, observance of diet-control is considered very essential for rectifying imbalance of *doṣas* which result in the emergence of diseases.

Diet, sleep and celibacy are considered as the three pillars of health. Diet is the primary source of life. Rāja Mānasollāsa suggests that the strength and lustre of one who knows the suitable diet and regimen for every season and practises accordingly are enhanced.[1] Enhancement of strength and lustre includes happiness, etc. resulting from maintaining equilibrium of tissue elements. The year is divided into six parts according to seasons. The northward movement of the sun and his act of evaporation bring about three seasons beginning from late winter to summer. The southward movement of the sun and the act of evaporation give rise to the other three seasons beginning with the rainy season.

It is not possible to have the knowledge about suitable diet and regimen for different seasons without having the knowledge about the seasons themselves. Even then, seasons are to be taken as separate entities. Taken together, they constitute the year inasmuch as the same seasons are repeated in rotation every year.

Classification of seasons for the purpose of administering five elimination therapies is different from the one described here. The following table furnishes a comparative view of the present classification :

According to Caraka such of the diets and regimens, as stand in contradistinction with the *doṣas* responsible for the production of the particular *prakṛti* (body constitution) are prescribed for the maintenance of positive health. For individuals, having equipoised state of *doṣas,* habitual intake of diets consisting of all *rasas* (tastes) in proportionate quantity is prescribed.[2]

रसs (*Rasas*)

The first of these, namely *rasa,* is a comprehensive term and needs some explanation. It does not mean 'taste' only as understood by the words "रसनार्थो रसस्तस्य"; it involves अनुरसs (*anu-rasas*) also which are detected by their effects on the system and which may not possess any taste. Pharmacologically, however, when its local action is taken into consideration, *rasa* means "direct action of a drug on the nerve-endings in the mucous membrane of the mouth." This action bears reference to the mechanism by which all rapid substances stimulate the gustatory nerves by means of their chemical constituents. Though no fixed theory regarding the association of any basic acid radical in a compound body with the creation of taste, has yet been formulated, it may do, for the sake of illustration, if we take it that the acids own their characteristic taste to H^+ ions in a compound, and that alkalies to their $(OH)^-$ ions.

In Āyurveda, all *dravyas,* whether organic or inorganic, are classified into six groups in accordance with their *rasa*-content. *Rasa* is taken as the basis, because it connotes a chemico-physical meaning. *Dravya,* of which *rasa* is only a part, is a support for पृथिवी and अप् *bhūtas* of which *āp-tatva* is the chief principle as it forms the source (योनिः) of the six *rasas.* So *āp-tatva* is a *karaṇa-dravya* and *rasa* is a *kārya-dravya.* Caraka says—"तेषां षण्णां रसानां योनिरुदकम्". He further continues to give reasons why only six *rasas* are to be considered in the evaluation of a *dravya.* Caraka says—

सौम्याः खल्वापोऽन्तरिक्षप्रभवाः पृकृतिशीता लघ्व्यश्चाव्यक्तरसाश्च, तास्त्वन्तरिक्षाद्भ्रश्यमाना भ्रष्टाश्च पंचमहाभूत गुणसमन्विता जङ्गमस्थावराणां भूतानां मूर्तिरभिप्रीणयन्ति, यासु मूर्तिषु षड्भिमूर्च्छन्ति रसाः ।।

(चरकसंहिता-सूत्रस्थान 26.37)

The *āpa-tatva,* which has descended to earth through आकाश (*ākāśa*), has its source in सोम (Soma). It is, therefore, cool and light by nature, and at the beginning of creation, its *rasa* is unmanifest, when, on its way downwards through *ākāśa,* It is influenced by the properties of the *pañcamahābhūtas.* It affects all the moveable and immovable objects in the world. And thus, it is that objects are endowed with the six *rasas* arising from the union.

These quotations indicate the physical constitution and the evolutionary source of *rasas.* The combinations of *Ap* and *Pṛthivī* are innumerable. Only some of them *vyakta-rasas,* while the other *Avyakta-rasas* or *anu-rasas*. The former are recognised immediately by the organ of taste, and the latter by their action on the constitution.

To complete the explanation that *rasa* has a comprehensive

range of action Caraka states[3]—

Rasa is the sense of taste residing in the tongue. पृथिवी and जल are its sources of development. The manifestation of *rasa* depends upon the properties of *ākāśa, vāyu* and *tejas,* and so too the creation of difference in taste (*rasa*).

The *vyakta-rasas* are only six. The *avyakta-rasas* are many. Hemadri is sufficiently clear on the differentiation between *rasa* and *anu-rasa.* He says, तत्रद्रव्ये, कश्चिद्धर्मः सद्योव्यक्तः, कश्चिदव्यक्तः, कश्चिदीषव्द्यक्तः, कश्चिदन्तेव्यक्तः। तेषु आद्योरसाख्यः, इतरे त्रयोऽनुरसाख्याः।।

Thus are formed the six *rasas.* The predominance of the elementary principles in each of them is given below :

Name of *rasa*					**Origin of *rasa***
1.	मधुर	—	*Madhura*	—	भूम्यंबुबाहुल्यात्
2.	आम्ल	—	*Āmla*	—	भूम्यग्निबाहुल्यात्
3.	लवण	—	*Lavaṇa*	—	तोयाग्निबाहुल्यात्
4.	कटु	—	*Kaṭu*	—	वाय्वग्निबाहुल्यात्
5.	तिक्त	—	*Tikta*	—	वाय्वाकाशबाहुल्यात्
6.	कषाय	—	*Kaṣāya*	—	पृथिव्यनिलबाहुल्यात्

It must be noted here that it is the *guṇas* of the *mahābhūtas* which represent the *rasas,* and not the *mahābhūtas* themselves. *Dravya* is only a common factor. In this connection Suśruta says[4]—

The relation between *rasa* and *dravya* (its support) is the same as that between the body and the soul; for they are both interdependent. On account of the chemical significance which *rasa* carries with it, Āyurvedists have adopted it as as standard for the classification of all drugs. The other properties of *dravyas* cannnot satisfy this purpose. *Guṇa* by itself is only a physical property, and being indefinite, it cannot be a unit for classification; *Vīrya* is described in terms of *guṇa,* but it works through *rasa,* for Caraka opines[5]—

Vipāka is virtually a *rasa* having undergone a transformation by digestive processes; and lastly, *prabhāva* is a specific property. Hence the importance of *rasa* both in therapeutics and in the classification of drugs. It can be stated in a nutshell that—

1. *Rasas* produce a direct or and immediate action, and the *aṇu-rasas,* an action which is not manifest.
2. The *rasas* have particular reference to the feeling of taste.
3. They produce an action on the mucous membranes, and even on the skin through the nerves.
4. The local action of *rasas* is availed of in therapeutical measures such as *swehana, swedana, nasya, basti,* etc.

Rasas belonging to *dravyas* are six in number. They are मधुर, आम्ल, लवण, तिक्त, उष्ण (कटु) and कषाय. The first is highly potent, while the others are proportionately less potent in a descending order. (अ.हृ.सू.अ. 1-14)

The prescription of diets consisting of all *rasas* in proper (same) quantity for individuals of *samaprakṛti* (having equipoised state of *doṣas*) needs further elucidation. It is not that all the *rasa* are intended to be taken in equal quantity. No healthy person will relish as much of pungent food as of sweet dishes. It will also not be helpful for the maintenance of health in the healthy person. So, the proportion of *rasas* is to be determined according to the individual's taste and food value. A *vāta-prakṛti* man may require more of diets having *madhura* (sweet), *āmla* (sour) and *lavaṇa* (saline) taste during winter, whereas for a *samaprakṛti* man, diets having all the tastes specially *āmla* (sour) and *lavaṇa* (saline) tastes are prescribed. Thus, the proportion of *rasa* is to be determined according to the bodily constitution (*prakṛti*), seasons, and dietetic property.—(*Aṣṭāṅgahṛdaya : Sūtra* 3 : 57).

Normally, mind, including sense faculties remains undisturbed. In order that they are not disturbed in any way, one should make all efforts to maintain their normal condition. This can be achieved by the performance of duties after duly considering their pros and cons with the help of intellect together with the sense faculties applied to their respective wholesome objects and in consideration with the qualities of place, season and one's own constitution including temperamemt. So one, who is desirous of his own well being should always perform noble acts with proper care.

The Rāja Mānasollāsa says, the normal condition of the sense faculties and mind can be maintained by certain therapeutic devices. Due performance of acts includes avoidance of harmful acts as well as performance of beneficial ones.[6]

Such efforts are conducive to the prevention of abnormal conditions of sense faculties and mind. If, on the other hand, the abnormal condition have already been created, they can be cured by acting, in contradistinction with the place, time and one's own constitution including temperament. So positive health can be maintained by due performance of acts as prescribed in scriptures. So, the one desirous of his own well-being should perform noble acts with proper care.

Rāja Mānasollāsa explains noble acts as follows :

One should pay respects to the Gods, cows, Brahmins, preceptors, elderly people, those who have accomplished spiritual perfection and teachers; one should offer oblation to the fire; one should perform *sandhyā* (a Vedic ritual to be performed during dawn, noon and dusk) thrice a day; one should clean excretory passages and feet frequently; one should have a hair cut, shave and and nail cut—thrice every fortnight; one should be happy, apply scent, wear good dress, comb the hair, always, apply oil to the head, ears, nostrils and feet, take initiative in wishing, have a dilightful face, protect people in affliction, offer oblation, perform religious ceremonies, give donations, offer *balis* (a religious oblation), honour the guests, offer *piṇḍas* (a ball or lump of rice offered to the manes [souls of the dead] at obsequial ceremonies or *śrāddhas),* to departed ancestors, speak timely beneficial, measured sweet words, be self-controlled and virtuous, engage in action but not in the results thereof, be careful and fearless, be bashful and wise, have enormous enthusiasm, be clever, forbearing, virtuous, having faith in God, devoted to teachers who have attained spiritual perfection and are advanced in modesty, intellect, learning, heredity and age; one should use an umbrella, a stick, a turban, shoes and see only six feet forward while walking; one should always acquit himself in an auspicious way and display good manners; one should avoid places with dirty appearance and strewn with bones, thorns, impure hair, chaff, garbage, ash, fragments of earthen vessels, stop exercise before exertion, be friendly to all creatures, reconcile the angry, console the frightened, be merciful to the poor, be truthful and be predominantly of compromising nature and tolerant towards unpalatable words uttered by others, be controller of intolerance, be of peaceful disposition and conquer the very roots of attachment and hatred.

A noble person should envy or have competitive spirit in so far as actions leading to prosperity or acquisition of knowledge are concerned. But one should never envy others' lot. That is to say, one should never wish others being deprived of prosperity, knowledge, etc. The fact, that one should be fearless, applies only to unavoidable causes of fear. If it is within one's capacity to overcome some fears, one should always be cautious so as to avoid facing the resultant situation. The act of being friendly to all creatures is to be taken in a universal sense. Even though, a physician may not be permitted to treat such of the patients as are charged with treason or are fallen otherwise, he should have inner sympathetic attitude towards them.

Food alone sustains life. Life loses all its charm without it. 'नास्त्याहारसमं सौख्यं' is a significant statement in 'शिवपुराणम्'. Food, properly taken, alone provides necessary strength, nutrition and contentment. It is mentioned in आयुर्वेद that eight-fold rules have to be kept in mind while taking food. They are—प्रकृति (nature), करण (processing), संयोग (combination), राशि (quantity), देश (place) and काल (time), भोक्ता (eater) and भोजन नियम (prescribed rules for taking food).[7]

About diet, Caraka opines that—One should eat in proper quantity. The quantity of food to be taken, again, depends upon the power of digestion (including metabolism).[8]

For maintenance of proper and positive health, one should first of all eat in proper quantity. Eating here includes all types of eatables which are taken by mouth.

Quantity to be eaten depends upon the power of digestion and metabolism. This, of course, applies to the eating of food and not of drugs; nor does it imply the extent of exercise one should resort to. Dosage of the drug, in fact, depends upon the seriousness of the disease as well as on the strength of the patient. Extent of exercise to be resorted to, is to be determined on the basis of the quantity of *doṣas* required to be eliminated and the degree up to which the power of digestion including metabolism is to be enhanced. Of course, care is to be taken so that there is no over-exertion or exhaution during the act of exercise. The power of digestion and metabolism, upon which depends the quantity of food intake, again varies according to the season as well the age of the individual. Thus, the quantity of food to be taken depends upon a number of factors.

Quantity of Food and Digestion

According to Rāja Mānasollāsa—(1.19.149 to 153) the amount of food which, without disturbing the equilibrium (of *dhātus* and *doṣas* of the body), gets digested as well as metabolised in proper time, is to be regarded as the proper quantity.[9] The relation of the quantity of food and the power of digestion and metabolism, needs some explanation. How shall we know that a given amount of food is just enough for a particular individual? This can be known only by correlating the food taken with its proper digestion within a time limit. If food taken in the evening does not disturb the equilibrium of *doṣas* as well as *dhātus* and gets digested and metabolised by the morning then that would be the standard quantum of food to be taken by the individual. This quantum varies from individual to individual. No standard quantum can be prescribed for all individuals. In fact, the power of digestion even of a single individual varies from time to time and so there is bound to be some variation in the standard quantum of food for an individual which is to be determined on the basis of his digestive capacity.

It is not that the food that gets digested in time may not disturb the equilibrium. It does so, owing to some inherent defects in its components, (premature curd), *lakuca (Artocarpus lakoocha* Roxb), etc. do disturb the equilibrium, irrespective of their quantity taken.

Measurement of food is in fact, of two types, viz., food as a whole and of its different ingredients having different tastes like sweet, sour, etc. If food as a whole is taken according to the prescribed measurement but its ingredients having different tastes like sweet, sour, etc., are not in prescribed ratio, the equilibrium of *dhātus* and *doṣas* gets definitely disturbed due to imbalance in the ratio of the composing *rasas* (tastes). Consequently the timely digestion of food as a whole, will also be affected.

According to *Caraka Saṁhitā*—मात्रावद्ध्यशनमशितमनुपहत्य प्रकृतिं बलवर्णसुखायुषा योजयत्युपयोक्तारमवश्यमिति ।। (चरकसंहिता-सूत्रस्थान ८)

Taken in appropriate quantity, food certainly helps the individual in bringing about strength, complexion, happiness and longevity without disturbing the equilibrium of *dhātus* and *doṣas* of the body.

Thus, the determination of the quantity of food depends upon the power of digestion and metabolism as well as the heaviness or lightness of the food articles concerned. Food taken in proper quantity, helps in bringing about the strength, complexion, happiness and longevity. Of course, there are other factors like inappropriateness of time, non-observance of ethical rules and unwholesomeness of auditory, tactile, visual, gustatory and olfactory sensations which might minimise the effects of taking wholesome food in proper time. But then other things being normal, food taken in proper quantity must do good to the body.

Caraka Saṁhitā opines[10] that—Good health stands at the very root of virtuous, acts acquirement of wealth, gratification of desire and final emancipation. Rāja Mānasollāsa states the same view—भाव्यं पथ्याशिना नित्यं नीरुजो जायते ततः। व्याधिभिर्वर्जितो राजा राजकार्य क्षमो भवेत्।। (2.1.10) Diseases are destroyers of health, well-being and life.

Dharma is associated with the soul itself which is to be inferred from its results. *Artha* is the attainment of wealth like gold, etc. *Kāma* is the fulfilment of desire like embracing women. *Mokṣa* is liberation from the world. *Ārogya,* i.e., health, represents the equilibrium of *dhātus* in the absence of diseases. Thus, health is the root cause *par excellence* of the attainment of all these four objects of human life inasmuch as one suffereing from a disease is absolutely incapable of performing any act conducive to the attainment of any of these four objects. As a matter of fact, the manifestation of diseases is synchronous with the impediments to the objects of human life. It is not correct to say that a disease is caused first and then it spoils health. The combination of a positive and a negative object would rather lead to a negative rather than a positive result. An impediment to the objects of human life, on the other hand, is to be treated as something positive rather than negative. Rāja Mānasollāsa opines that—life without happiness is not worth living. Conversely, life with happiness alone is worth living.

After keeping in mind the above prescriptions, one should take food so as to avoid any possible disorders. It is also necessary to take food after the previous meal is digested and real appetite demands it. It is not easy for others to determine whether anybody is hungry. Each has to know whether he/she is really hungry. क्षुधा—hunger, if genuine, is a sign of good health. Want of क्षुधा or loss of appetite is a symptom of disorder or disease. It is for this very reason that diet is considered as one of the pillars of health. Āyurveda prescribes diet-restriction—पथ्य as a must and so physicians always advise to avoid अद्यशन—over-eating, विषमाशन—irregular eating and समशन—mixed eating. Any food taken before the previous meal is digested is called अद्यशन. Irregularity in respect of quantity and time is considered विषमाशन. When wholesome and unwholesome items are mixed together it is called समशन. These three are known as perversions of eating and one would do well to avoid them.[11]

It is considered advisable to keep a gap of three hours before two meals. If one eats earlier, it causes indigestion. Late meals always result in weakness. This relates to time-gap in taking food. Even regarding quantity to be consumed, there are rules to be followed strictly. If the diet consists of two parts of solid and one part of liquid, it is considered very ideal. The remaining part or one quarter is better to be kept vacant in the stomach. This is necessary because it facilitates easy movement of *doṣas.*[12]

It is necessary to keep in mind the fact that barring a few common substances, articles of food vary from climate to climate and place to place. This in turn necessitates change in food habits of people living in different climates. This results in the consumption of vegetarian and non-vegetarian dishes. Rice, wheat and vegetables may be considered as common everywhere. They are items of stable food also. Pulses are also used as food for human beings and feed for cattle. Normally a smaller percentage of the people are purely vegetarians whereas the majority supplement the diet with meat. Use of intoxicant drinks and juices are also common. King Someśvara is all praise for good food prepared by expert cooks. Good food is essential for nourishment and maintenance of health. Good food served with love acts as a tonic. Even scholars in the west agree on this point—"Good food is a symbol of love, having psychological value which may even exceed its sensory and physiological contributions."[13]

Instructions regarding proper preparation of some food items are found in Rāja Mānasollāsa. It is remarkable that Someśvara had time and patience to observe this aspect of life also minutely. The detailed description of the preparation of पायस, मण्डक, पीलिका, पूरिका, दोसका, इड्डरिका, घारिका, वटिका etc., bear testimony to the fact that he was also an expert who knew the art of cooking and selection of noted items in the diet.

Preparation of non-vegetarian dishes has also not missed Someśvara's attention. He suggests mild fire or low temperature heat as most suitable in preparing meat dishes. Details of preparing several non-vegetarian dishes are given in third *Prakaraṇa* of chapter 13 *Annopabhogya,* in Rāja Mānasollāsa. This is corroborated by western experts also on cookery. Adelle Davis says on this point—Meat should be cooked at low temperature. There are many advantages in cooking meat at low temperature. At low temperature meats shrink a little and they become juicier and more delicious.[14]

Rāja Mānasollāsa mentions how congenial it is to change dishes and drinks in accordance with the need of different seasons. "Pungent things in spring, sweet and cold things in summer, salty things in rainy season, sweet things in autumn, greasy and hot things in early winter and sour things in late winter are most suited for health."[15] This is in accordance with the prescription of Āyurveda. It also mentions that butter-milk after lunch, milk after dinner and water early in the morning are very beneficial drinks for maintaining good health.

Food is the main stay of life. But the same thing consumed without discrimination becomes poison, harming life. Dishes prepared out of milk are tasty. Without ghee it is tasteless. Food with ghee, soup and thick curds are most welcome. Food without meat is not relished by many. Varieties of dishes are enjoyed by one and all. Taste alone is not the criterion in diet. It must be wholesome and healthy and nourishing as well. Harmless and easily digestable food is always welcome. Balanced diet, taken in time, is the best for maintaining health. Irregular food causes painful diseases and so the physician always prescribes a healthy, limited and timely diet and advises the patient to be wary of being tempted by taste. Over-eating and undue fasting also are to be avoided even by a healthy person, what to speak of a patient. Only food digested gets assimilated as आहाररस discarding the unassimilated portion as मल.

Drugs prove efficacious only when the patient is looked after by the attendants providing him/her with proper nourishing diet. Time-gap, quantity to be consumed, quantum of solid and liquid contents etc., have to be strictly observed by the attendants who are in charge of the ailing patient. In short, medication along with nursing with love helps in restoring the normal physical and mental health of a patient. Encouraging response from the patient's side makes the physician attending on him to be more enthusiastic in helping him for steady and speedy recovery.

Looking at the slow improvement of the patient, the physician allows him/her orderly exercises.

Drug, diet and activity form the main factors in this course of restoration of normal health. Drug is prescribed after proper diagnosis and thorough testing. Diet is advised as a suitable nourishment both for the body and the mind. Activity is suggested to suit the requirement of the patient to recover as early as possible. It is worth remembering here that the pan of a balance bends too low with heavy weight. With light weight, it goes up. With equal weight on either-side, it maintains balance. Similarly, the body with normal diet and activity can respond to the drug effectively.

यथाभारेण नमते लघुनोन्नमते तुला।
समातिष्ठति युक्तेन भोज्येनेयं तथा तनुः।।
तस्मादभ्यवहर्तव्यं स्वशक्तिमनुपश्यता।
नातिपात्रं च नात्यल्पं मेयं मानवशादपि।।

(सौन्दरानन्द[16])

A normally healthy person can satisfy realise his/her hunger and take suitable diet. He/she can also decide upon the quantity he/she has to take. But a diseased person cannot do so. He/she has to depend on the persons attending on him/her who are advised by the physician treating him/her. These attendants have to remember that जठराग्नि, gastric fire, of a patient is dormant. As the process of पाक—digestion and transformation depend upon जठराग्नि, the patient has to be under liquid or solid diet according to the interval or time-gap suggested by the physician. It is also necessary for the attendant to watch not only the intake of प्रसार or essence for nourishment, but also the time of evacuation or excreta or मल and urine मूत्र of the patient. They are also to give authentic report of the colour of urine and hard or smooth evacuation of excreta. The quantity of urine and stool evacuated has also to be brought to the notice of the physician. मल evacuated periodically helps the body of the patient to assimilate रस. मल stuck up defiles the body and the patient cannot relish any dish in that state. Drugs also will not yield the desired result.

अग्नि is the invariable agent in the process of धातुपाक—metabolism. आयुर्वेद mentions three types of अग्नि-जठराग्नि, भूताग्नि and धात्वग्नि. जठराग्नि is gastric fire also known as वैश्वनर. This is present in all living beings. This is essential for digestion of food. It transforms food into रस and मल. भूताग्नि is expected to act upon the *bhautika* portion of food and nourish the पंचभूतs. धात्वग्नि acts upon the धातुs. Each धातु is of three types. The gross part is मल to be evacuated. The fine part remains as it is. The finer one helps in the formation of धातु.[17]

As the patient has delicate physique, this अग्नि which is very active in the process of पाक, digestion and transformation, is below normal in heat. So digestion is not easy and transformation is slow. In order to activate them, the physician resorts to extra-drugs and determines their dosage required for the purpose. This is brought to the notice of the attendants who have to strictly adhere to the instruction and help the patient to regain his stamina and build up resistance.

It is worth remembering at this stage that वात, पित्त and कफ when aggravated, cause all disorders and diseases. These aggravated *doṣas* need to be pacified by the prescribed drug and diet. Soothing substances and intake of sweet and salty-sour items are known for pacifying वात. *Pitta* gets pacified with sweets, bitters and astringents and intake and sprinkling of cold water. Bitter, astringent and pungent substances bring down कफ. Even after the acute disorder or disease is brought under control and normalcy is restored, patients's state of health remains delicate. At such a crucial stage, even the slightest negligence regarding drug and diet intake on the part of the patient, is harmful. There is every chance of relapse. Therefore, the attendant has to exercise great tact in persuading the patient to resist all temptation for delicious dishes in the diet. The physician also gives the patient a mild warning and advises him to be visiting him for observation. Āyurvedic treatment is a little harsher in regard to पथ्यापथ्य as compared to the allopathic treatment. But one should always remember that Āyurvedic treatment always aims at curing an ailment and not merely preventing or suppressing it.

Our ancient literature has given some information about digestion and health. Some general statements on the subject are quoted below[18] :

1. Even after a lapse of a long time, the following do not harm a person; well-digested food; a very smart son; a

well-disciplined wife; a beneficient ruler; a well thought-provoking speech and a methodical action.[19]

2. One, who takes food after the earlier food is properly digested, does not contract any disease.[20]
3. Disturbed study is harmful for learning. Soiled clothes spoil the beauty of a woman. Proper digestion of food wards off diseases. Exhibition of prowess weakens an enemy.[21]
4. A fool does not begin to work being afraid of faulting. My dear friend! Does any one stop eating being afraid of food causing indigestion?[22]
5. Normally, irregular food causes indigestion. Diseases crop up due to indigestion. Diseases vanish when the cause of indigestion is stopped.[23]
6. Improper learning, undigestible food, gossipping by a poor man, a young wife for an aged person, all these are injurious like poison.[24]
7. If unhealthy food once taken is not digested properly, one should not take even a healthy food.[25]

'आर्यावर्तः पुण्यभूमिः' is not a mere slogan, but a reality for those inhabiting this vast land from times immemorial. It is also a homeland for those who have sought shelter here being driven out of their native land for reasons beyond their control. Both the original inhabitants and those subsequently finding this as their homeland, considered it their privilege to have been born or found shelter here. It is a पुण्यभूमि for those born here. But the greatness of this land is acknowledged by the new settlers as पुण्यभूमि. That is why this acquires significance when you proclaim आर्यवर्त as पुण्यभूमि. It is sacred because this land is the home of आर्यs—cultured or most humane. Nowhere one comes across the life-sustaining inspiration as is reflected in the pithy saying—

'सर्वेभवन्तु सुखिनः सर्वे सन्तु निरामयाः'

'May all be happy and may all be free from ill-health.'

Indians are proud of having a chain of Rulers who considered the well-being of their subjects as their mission and a galaxy of physicians who saw to it that all were made aware of the importance of health—mental, moral and physical and guarding against any contamination, both internal and external. When viewed in this context, Rāja Mānasollāsa of King Someśvara III of the Cālukya dynasty of Karnataka, stands as an immortal piece of Sanskrit literature covering all aspects of human aspirations.

Rāja Mānasollāsa is considered an encyclopaedia. Dr. M.M. Kalburgi, former Vice-chancellor of Hampi University, has rightly observed that there are four encyclopaedias which have opened a grand vista before the Kannadigas where they can have a glimpse of their rich cultural heritage. *Lokopakāra* of Caundarāya and *Vivekacintāmaṇi* of Nijaguna Shivayogi are in Kannada language. *Śivatattwa Ratnākara* of Keladi Basava Bhoopala and Rāja Mānasollāsa of Someśvara are in Sanskrit. Someśvara was the son of Vikramāditya VI. Kalyāṇa was the capital of Cālukya dynasty. Vikramāditya VI is regarded as a collossus in Karnataka history who ruled over Kalyāṇa for nearly five decades. His son Someśvara III, unlike other princes, made the best use of his leisure in bringing out Rāja Mānasollāsa which is a culmination of self-revelation based on minute study and keen observation.

Rāja Mānasollāsa has for its inspiration Kauṭilya's अर्थशास्त्र, Kamandaka's नीतिसार, Hemacandra's लघ्वर्थ नीतिशास्त्र, and Bhoja's शालिहोत्र. One may include अग्निपुराण and मत्स्यपुराण also in this list. These sources have enabled Someśvara to rise above the regional calculations and view life in a larger perspective. In these days of globalisation and liberalisation when barriers have no meaning, the world view of Someśvara attracts universal attention. 'Think globally and act locally' seems to have been his motto and perhaps this emboldened him to write in Sanskrit.

'Rāja Mānasollāsa' is considered as a product of the 12th

century in Karnataka where there was a great renaissance and reformation. This was a period when tradition was being questioned both at the level of thought and expression. A new cult was shaping itself storming the citadel of the old and a new language was being employed to awaken the masses. It is amazing to see Someśvara remaining firm and unruffled by this storm around him and restate the eternal values for a changing society in his immortal Rāja Mānasollāsa in Sanskrit. It is, therefore, appropriate that this classic work is known by the title '*Rāja Mānasollāsa*', '*Abhilāṣitārtha Cintāmaṇi*' etc.

A physician, worth the name, is also expected to be thoroughly acquainted with the environment, such as seasonal variations and cleanliness or otherwise of the surroundings where the patient is undergoing treatment or convalescing for, proper diagnosis and prescribing treatment, 'देश'—habitat, and काल—time, are very important. Diet restrictions are also very essential. So, a chapter detailing the environmental factors governing the upkeep of the body and its capacity for resistance is included.

Āyurveda course of treatment imposes diet restrictions for the prescribed drugs for benefiting the patient. पथ्य-अपथ्य, भक्ष्य-अभक्ष्य, पेय-अपेय are, therefore, suggested by the physician. If the ailing person strictly follows the suggestion in letter and spirit, a steady and slow recovery is assured. Otherwise, it may prove very fatal also. No wonder-drug prescribed by even a धन्वंतरि can achieve the desired end if the diseased person ignores the physician's suggestions regarding पथ्य, भक्ष्य and पेय.

Rāja Mānasollāsa of Someśvara III is a unique contribution for a cultural study of Āyurveda as well as other sources of knowledge to make life worth living. Modern medicine lays stress on all types of Tests—blood, urine, stool, etc. It is in medical parlance known as blood-culture, urine-culture and stool-culture. This is supposed to give a clue on the basis of which a physician bases his diagnosis and determines the course of treatment. Āyurveda lays emphasis on नाडिपरीक्षा pulse-examination to find the condition of the constitution of an ailing person. According to Āyurveda, the health of an individual depends solely on the maintenance of the routine according to his constitution. At the same time, the physician is required to keep the constitution of the ailing person in mind before prescribing any medicine and advising diet-restriction.

There is no gainsaying the fact that only when the patient is responsive to the timely treatment of the physician, much of the mishap can be averted. At the same time, if the physician is sympathetic in understanding the patient and is efficient in suggesting suitable remedies, things can click. Any callousness on the part of a physician and negligence on the part of a patient spoils the Āyurvedic course of treatment.

It is said that faith is continuation of reason. Only faith in the process of diagnosis and prescription of right medicine at the right moment on the part of a physician can ward off risks in treatment. Only faith in the physician on the part of a patient can help him/her to revoer fast and gain his/her normal health.

Modern medicine with all the hitech equipments at its command like X-ray, shock-treatment, by-pass surgery, bone-setting, contact-lenses, laser treatment, hearing-aids, etc., has only made treatment very expensive and beyond the reach of the have nots. Only VIPs with Government patronage and expenses can avail of all facilities. We are not decrying the utility of these things. But it cannot be anything other than a sad commentary, when ailing persons have to go in search of Nursing Homes not only in urban areas but also in rural zones for securing proper attention involving exorbitant costs.

In this context, the treatment of the state of a physician in a progressive society depicted in Rāja Mānasollasa by Someśvara III makes a refreshing study. How far this is going to make an impact on the minds of those that matter in the present day society remains to be seen.

Significance of Physicians

Rājā or the king is essential for the welfare of the people, who in the remote past had realised his importance for the protection of their social and economic institutions. The people were unsafe without a ruling authority to hold and inflict the *Daṇḍa* upon those who did not follow the rule of law. A King is the root cause of all success and happiness. He creates spiritual atmosphere by protecting the *Dharma. Rājā* is the person, who encourages the development of arts and culture in his kingdom. He is, therefore, essential for the all-round development of the people.

Someśvara throws a flood of light on the contemporary social ideals. The administration of social justice is one of the most important functions to be discharged by the State. The *Daṇḍa* is a coercive but an effective power given to the king for regulating the life of the subjects. The State is not an idle institution; it is not an onlooker of the happenings, but is a forceful and living institution to correct those persons who do not follow the rules of conduct, either established by tradition or prescribed by scriptures.

The Rāja Mānasollāsa regards *Dharma* as the root of the State. Hence, the enforcement of law or *Daṇḍa* is essential for its existence.[26] The *Maryādā* or moral law is well established in society when the king controls the evils and shows compassion towards the virtuous.[27]

Medicine is given a place of pride in Atharvaṇa Veda. It was believed that the words of the priests possessing knowledge of medicine were thought to bring them into direct contact with the greater cosmic forces. The healers also required knowledge of the means to control the natural forces in order to set right again what had gone wrong in the first place. Combining their expertise in accessing and manipulating the spiritual world with the knowledge they acquired from the sacrificial cults, the healers became the priests of the third estate, operating along with the sacrificial priests of the first estate. The roles of each type of priests were quite distinct, but outwardly they probably resembled each other in many respects.

The medical priest probably enjoyed relatively more freedom in the social structure and was not confined to a particular social group, as he served the needs of all people regardless of their social standing. The sacrificial priest, on the other hand, fearing contamination and from impure elements of the society, was restricted to the milieu (social surroundings) of the first order. It would not be unreasonable to assume that competition between priests for power and prestige may well have emerged. With time, the healers became recognized by their counterparts in the first estate as contaminating and eventually being excluded from the higher, more sacred circles of the sacrificial cults. They were gradually forced to remain in their own communities of the third estate, located at the margins of society where contact with many sorts of people with different healing traditions might well have taken place. This removal of healers and their special craft from the main stream Vedic priestly culture led eventually to a radical shift in medical thinking.

Rājadharma, according to Rāja Mānasollāsa, was the foundation for the well-being of a society in ancient India. The welfare of the society was considered as the primary responsibility of a king.. The king was expected to provide all facilities for the people belonging to various strata or categories. A kingdom can prosper and make rapid progress only when the ruler helps in regulating the life of his subjects in accordance with rules of conduct as established by tradition and prescribed by scriptures which constitute Rājadharma.

Maintenance of a standard administration, conducive to social justice, was considered as a sacred religious duty of a king. Any violation of scriptural sanctions invited serious punishment to the ruler as well as the subjects ruled by him. Such an eventuality could be avoided only by the enforcement of moral law established in society in accordance with *Varṇāśramadharma.* This would help in upholding the cause of justice and rewarding virtue. It would also control, if not eliminate, injustice and evil. People do not normally deviate from scriptural injunctions when their king is the guardian of his subjects, administering justice impartially and keeping them contented by providing all facilities in their day-to-day work. Unrest and disorder spread in a society when there is a clash of interests among individuals or groups. This can be avoided when the principles common to all the four *Āśramas* are scrupulously observed in letter and spirit by all. Non-injury, truthfulness, non-wickedness and forgiveness are some of these common principles. The king has to regulate the affairs of the state in a manner when everyone performs his or her rightful duties or *Svadharma* without any hindrance. It is the duty of the king to extend protection to all in the performance of their duties or *Svadharma.* In order to ensure social harmony and public safety, the king appoints a large number of officers to enforce law and order.

Rāja Mānasollāsa discusses in detail the nature of *Svadharma* of the four *Āśramas. Brahmacarya* (celibacy), *Grastya* (house-holder's duty), *Vānaprastha* (retiring to the forest) and *Sanyāsa* (life of a recluse) are the four *Varṇas* or *Āśramas.* Studying of the Vedas, performing ablutions at prescribed time, staying with the preceptor or teacher till the end of the student life, living on alms and worshipping fire are the duties of a *Brahmachāri.* Earning livelihood by proper means, marrying among equals, living in harmony with wife and children and making gifts form the duties of a householder. Observance of continence and living on the forest produce are the duties of a *Vānaprastha.* Purity, both external and internal, with strict control of the senses is the hallmark of a *Sanyāsi.* The king is assisted by his officers in helping his subjects to fulfil their *Svadharma.*

Attendants, cooks, palace guards, superintendents of the various departments and family physician form the king's personal staff. Apart from these, there are officers who are under the direct control of the king. Rāja Mānasollāsa makes a special mention of *Dharmādhikāris* or judges who help the king in administering justice.

Ministers appointed by the king act as advisers of the ruler in policy-making matters. Army commanders are there to look after the military affairs and security of the state. Judicial officers or *Dharmadhikāris* ensure speedy and efficient justice. Revenue officers are entrusted with the task of collecting and fair distribution of revenue among the various departments. Economic prosperity of the state depends upon their proper and timely discharge of duties. A group of wise men advise the king on religious matters.

Educationists and specialists in cultural affairs look after the promotion of education and culture.

It is the duty of a shrewd king to identify the honest and selfless officers and entrust responsibilities to them. The king has to be very vigilant. A just and benevolent king enjoys the loyalty of his officers who love to render honest and efficient service to the state under the ruler. Honest and efficient officers are also respected and honoured by the king. The king encourages such loyal officers by praise and presents, and keeps them contented. A trustworthy group of officers is an asset to the state, both for the king and his subjects. In this respect, the king has to be very alert and keep himself at a safe distance from his ministers and officers. Someśvara agrees with Somadeva who in his यशस्तिलक mentions how a king is taken unawares by his over smart officers. Somadeva says, "kings who enjoy pleasures at will, leaving the charge of the kingdom in the hands of officers, are indeed foolish. They might as well go to sleep leaving the cats in charge of the milk. The movement of fish in water and birds in the sky might sometimes be known, but the conduct of the ministers, inscrutable, impalpable unvouchable matters can never be known."[28]

The duties and responsibilities of the different categories of officers of the king are dealt within detail in कामन्दकीय नीतिसार, Kauṭilya's अर्थशास्त्र, Somadeva's यशस्तिलक, Bhoja's युक्तिकल्पतरु and other works. Someśvara has followed them in Rāja Mānasollāsa in describing the duties and qualifications of officers of the king.

Someśvara lays emphasis on foreign relations in the state administration. He considers the status of a *Dūta* or an envoy as very important. A *Dūta* or an envoy should be well-versed in all Arts and Sciences. He should be amiable and unruffled in the face of severe provocation. Manu extols the role of an envoy in the following words :

"Let him also appoint the *Dūta* who is well-versed in all branches of knowledge, who is quick in understanding gestures and expressions of the face, who is honest, skillful and of a noble family. Such an ambassador or envoy is commended to a king."[29]

Similarly, the role of the spies in the set-up is very significant. A spy is regarded as a second sight for the king. From the time of Manu, the institution of espionage is considered a very significant unit of the administration. Manu states–

"Having performed twilight-oblations, let him well-armed, hear in an inner apartment, the doings of those who make secret reports and of his spies."[30]

Yājñavalkya also mentions about the king attentively listening to the secret report—गूढ़भाषितम्—submitted by the spies.

Whenever the king comes to know of the wrong doings of his civil servants, he must exercise caution in inflicting punishment on the guilty only after sifting the grain from the husk. The king has to satisfy himself personally about the nature of such lapses before arriving at any decision. He should not rely only on the information given to him by his assistants in determining the quantum of punishment to be meted out to the culprits. He should not be unduly harsh in dispensing justice. No offence should go unpunished. At the same time, the king must keep in mind the fact that the guilty must be allowed a chance to clarify his/her stand and prove his/her innocence before pronouncing him/her guilty. In case the king fails to do so, 'he will be guilty of finding fault in an innocent person or he may allow the guilty to go unpunished. Under such circumstances he stands ridiculed and loses his credibility.' (मानसोल्लास:).[31] Nature of crime should determine the mild or severe punishment. According to Someśvara 'दोषानुरूपदंडत्व'—Punishment according to guilt, raises the concept of *Dharma* and *Daṇḍa*. The concept of *Dharma* is the basic foundation for understanding any judicial system. *Dharma* is a way of life. It is not mere 'religion'. This is no rigid system. It is ever changing and is the determining factor of moral law. This codified moral law is sustained by values which are deep rooted in this way of life. This is protected and preserved by a benevolent ruler who enforces its observance by the people of the state. The observance of these values by the subjects, helps in evolving the social and moral principles governing the conduct and behaviour of the people. This regulates the duties and responsibilities of the members of a society cultivating in *Āśramas* or *Varṇa Dharma*. It is the duty of the king to direct the people to observe these duties. Violation of *Dharma* invites punishment as decided by the king. In short, *Dharma* stands for moral and ethical values governing a civilized society where men and women are free to perform their chosen duties under the guidance of a wise king.

Equally important is the concept of *Daṇḍa* which means the symbol of royal authority to enforce discipline on the people under his jurisdiction of the state. Evolution of an egalitarian society and maintenance of peace are possible only when the king judiciously exercises the authority derived from *Daṇḍaneeti*—(दण्डनीति). *Daṇḍa* is the last among the four means recommended by all law givers and Someśvara III adheres to this—

उपायत्रितयेनापि यो न शक्यो भवेद्रिपुः।
तस्य दंडं प्रयुञ्जीत बलवान् यदि भूपतिः।। 2-20-1031

(When the other three means fail to control the enemy, a powerful ruler has to resort to the means of *Daṇḍa).*

Rāja Mānasollāsa enumerates fifteen types of *Daṇḍa* to curb the indiscipline of the rowdy elements in a state and the king has the inherent right to employ them as and when needed. The king can put down the anti-social elements by eliminating their hamlets and hideouts, amputating any of their organs, depriving them and their accomplices of their means of livelihood and physically eliminating them for their heinous crime.[32] Administering prisons through various means, causing fatal injuries to the enemy and adoption of sorcery had been legitimised during Someśvara's time. As a last resort, *Daṇḍa* is permissible for the preservation of *Dharma* which alone can protect the all-round prosperity of an individual or a group in a society and promote a steady progress of a state.

Religion occupies a place of pride under *Dharma.* Although *Dharma* is equated with religion in common parlance, it is not mere religion. Religion is a main plank under *Dharma.* Rāja Mānasollāsa emphasises the importance of religion, religious faith and religious practices in a society and a king is enjoined by scriptures to promote all religious practices strictly according to *Dharma.* The Hindu *Dharma* is based on श्रुति, स्मृति, सदाचार and परंपरा. These are the four perennial sources of *Dharma.*

श्रुति is the group of Vedas which are direct revelations of truth and higher truth narrated in the form of stories meant for the common people. सदाचार is upright conduct of virtuous people not opposed to the rules formulated by श्रुति and स्मृति। सदाचार is upright conduct gradually resulting in the growth of customs regulating community living. परंपरा or tradition according to

Manu comprises of देश—Local habitation, जाति—Caste, कुल—family or race and श्रेणी—category.[33]

कुलधर्म evolves according to religious rituals and helps in developing family traditions or customs. जातिधर्म constitutes customs and practices peculiar to different castes and sub-castes. Someśvara is the most broadminded king when he says, 'God is one. Do not hate any God.'[34]

देशधर्म is the product of a local habitation of a particular race. This is not necessarily followed throughout a country. देशधर्म is responsible for many diversifications in Hindu laws and customs in different regions. It is the duty of a ruler to protect and promote different social customs practised and propagated by different वर्णs and आश्रमs. Preservation of this order is the primary responsibility of a king.

Rāja Mānasollāsa strictly adheres to the *Dharma śāstra* and does not plead for any disturbance in the accepted norm.

Social customs gain currency through the संस्कारs as embodied in the *Śāstras.* Rāja Mānasollāsa discusses in detail the merits and importance of all the relevant संस्कारs and advocates the strict performance of the same. '*Garbhādhāna, Pumsavana, Sīmantonnayana, Jātakarma, Nāmakaraṇa, Annaprāśana, Karṇavedha, Cūdākarma, Upanayana, Godāna, Vivāha* etc., are elaborated in Rāja Mānasollāsa for a prince.'[35]

There are a number of rites and practices advocated by Someśvara to obtain occult (super-natural) power for miraculous effects. It is amusing to note the recipes recommended for handsome appearance in old age, possessing दिव्यशरीर, ability to disappear—अदृश्य, attaining longevity to move in space—आकाश, remaining without food for days together and walking long distances without getting tired. Various types of *vanaspathi* or herbal medicines to achieve such miraculous effects are described by him.

Someśvara's minute observation is revealed in his treatment of widespread belief in various omens and portents in the lives of individuals and groups. Both auspicious and inauspicious omens are described by him. Interpreting the significance of dreams is another attraction in Rāja Mānasollāsa. Belief in astrological predictions is mentioned in the work. Palmistry also was studied and practised during those days. Popular belief in planets and the various astronomical conjunctions and their good and bad effects on the destiny of living beings is a source of rich entertainment in Rāja Mānasollāsa.

Subjects relating to rites and practices of popular religion which moulded the socio-cultural pattern of the society during Someśvara's time, are also discussed in Rāja Mānasollāsa.

Temporal life was never neglected by him. Importance of regulated food and drinking habits conducive to health and beauty is also emphasised by the king. Someśvara does not ignore the niceties of vegetarian and non-vegetarian dishes prepared by expert cooks. Dinner and cock-tail parties were the order of the day during celebrations of birth day, marriage in the families and meetings, sports and games in society at large.

Amusements and entertainments reflected the tastes of urban and rural people of his times. Varieties of socio-cultural festivals provided opportunities for the exhibition of talents in various arts and literary field. Periodical meetings conducted by the literary and artistic associations are highlighted in Rāja Mānasollāsa. The various types of excursions organised by the people helped them to relax and enjoy rich social life. The importance of *Goṣtis* or meetings during those times connected with different types of learning, art and literature, reflects the cultural enrichment of the people. *Goṣtis* were varied in their composition. *Śāstragoṣtis* were related to the discussion on the scriptures. *Vidagdhagoṣtis* comprised of members of creative imagination and profound learning. *Kathāgoṣtis* stressed the importance of ornate *Kāvya* style. *Saṅgītagoṣtis* encouraged musical concerts. All these *goṣtis* were patronised by the king who participated occasionally along with his nobles in them. Someśvara himself an authority on music took keen interest in musicology and vocal and instrumental music. Music and dance received special encouragement and people participated in these *goṣtis* in large numbers.

Besides the various periodical *goṣtis* described above, performance of acrobatic feats and magicians and snake-charmers formed other sources of entertainment.

Swinging was very popular among ladies. The king had arranged for mechanical swings in the palace gardens and the ruler enjoyed swinging with his consorts in the spring season.

Rāja Mānasollāsa refers to many types of animal fighting and bird fighting which formed additional sources of entertainment. Special mention is made of a variety of elephant-fighting and horse-fighting, cock-fighting, Lāvaka-fighting, pigeon-fighting, etc. Hunting was another popular sport and source of entertainment. The vivid description of all these entertainments show how keen king Someśvara was in maintaining standard entertainments for himself and for his subjects.

Rāja Mānasollāsa gives a detailed description of the institution of marriage in a society. Someśvara's keen insight is astonishing when he prescribes qualifications and features of brides and grooms during the time of selection.

Someśvara is a champion of proper education for creating awareness among the people to dedicate themselves for building a strong and progressive welfare state. Ignorance is the root cause of all evils in a society. Knowledge and learning serve as a beacon light in removing the thick veil of darkness. Someśvara is fully conscious of the utility of a properly planned system of education. He had realised that the lamp of learning illuminates the course of worldly life making it smooth and happy. He was a protagonist of *Gurukula* system of education where the learned and an enlightened *Kulapathi* shaped the younger generation to develop a healthy mind in a healthy body. Pupils from far off places came to *Gurukulas* to receive training under eminent scholars in different branches of study. The king patronised such learned men with sterling character by making liberal grants and endowments in the form of *Agrahāras. Agrahāra,* according to G.S. Dikshit 'was a grant from the king to an individual or group of individuals, preferably householders, engaged in acquiring knowledge and devoted to the spread of learning."[36]

A teacher of an Agrahāra was held in high esteem by the king. A teacher was also addressed as *Guru, Āchārya, Upādhyāya* in Rāja Mānasollāsa. The relationship of a pupil and preceptor was based on love and service. According to Someśvara, *Gurukulas* were not only the centres of learning but were also centres for promoting culture and civilization. Acquisition of knowledge and spread of learning, both secular and spiritual, were the hallmarks of *Gurukulas.*

Art and architecture form the rich cultural heritage of any country. Paintings, pictures, monuments form the glorious contribution of the people. There is an extensive and exhaustive survey of these achievements in Rāja Mānasollāsa. It shows how Someśvara was a keen student and admirer of the cultural enrichment of his period. He patronised the growth and development of art in his kingdom.

Someśvara was an erudite scholar and closely watched the progress of science in the land. Astronomy and mathematics had greatly developed in ancient India and through the Greeks and Arabs it spread to the whole world. Indians assimilated the new approach to the subject introduced by outside contact. Rāja Mānasollāsa gives a detailed description of the advancement of science in the field of mathematics and study of planets.

The application of science has been playing a very important part in our daily life. Some people are wonderstruck by the tricks science can do, and they would like to know how these remarkable powers have been developed. Such information is probably even more important than a knowledge of the result of science. What was the 'last word' on some subjects a year ago, may have been left behind by today. These changes in the scientific field are puzzling the layman who thinks that once something is 'discovered' or 'proved', nothing can alter it. A study of the history of science shows that its results are true only within specific limits. When we can state fairly and exactly the conditions under which a particular result will be obtained, we can be confident of applying it under such circumstances. This is a part of all the methods of science.

In ancient India, astronomy, astrology and mathematics formed the three main divisions of *Jyotiṣa.* The movements of planets were studied from very early period and their influence on the weather, the plant life and human life was also recognised and studied. This resulted in the development of astronomy and astrology. Calculations of the movements of the celestial bodies and working out their positions gave rise to the science of mathematics.

The *Bṛhatsaṁhita* in 106 chapters deals with astrology, geography, weather, characteristic marks on the bodies of men, women, etc., omens and many such things. Pṛthuyasas, son of Varāhamihira, is the author of *Horāṣaṭpañcāśikā,* which along with the work of his father has been commented upon by Bhaṭṭotpala of the 10th century A.D. In the year 1172 A.D., the great mathematician Bhāskarācārya wrote the *Siddhānta-śiromaṇī* consisting of four parts—(1) *Līlāvatī,* (2) *Bījagaṇitaṁ,* (3) *Grahagaṇitaṁ* and (4) *Gola.* Astronomy and medicine are the two branches of science, the development of which started with the dawn of civilization. The curiosity about the heavenly bodies and their movements prompted the ancient mankind to become stargazers.

With the advance of time the treatment of the subject has undergone far reaching changes. Accordingly Science of medicine and treatment of various types of diseases received steady attention at the hands of Indian physicians. Someśvara praises the role of physicians in diagnosis and cure of both physical and psychological ailments. Āyurveda was a subject of deep study by Indian physicians. Rāja Mānasollāsa has made a thorough survey of theoretical and practical knowledge of this subject and has helped society to improve the health of the people and increase their longevity. As science of life, Āyurveda is considered as a supplement to Vedas. Eminent innovators in the line are Caraka and Suśruta who have left a deep impression on this branch upgrading it as *Upaveda* of Atharvaveda. The elevation of this branch of science from the physical to the spiritual plain is a great contribution of Caraka.

Someśvara has referred to almost all the texts on Indian medicine. The epithet of *Aṣtaṅga* indicates the analytical mind of the practitioners of Indian medicince.[37] Vāgbhaṭa's *Aṣṭāṅgahṛdaya, Carakasaṁhitā* by Agniveśa and *Suśruta-saṁhitā* by Suśruta are the main authoritative sources on Indian medicine. Both healthy and sick persons can benefit by the methods of treatment recommended by Agniveśa in *Caraka-saṁhitā*. Rāja Mānasollāsa is also considered as a very useful source of information for physicians, teachers, researchers and students of Āyurveda.

A thorough knowledge of the fundamental principles of Āyurveda and systematic practice of its eight specialised branches is very necessary for a physician. The nineteenth chapter of the first *prakaraṇa* in Rāja Mānasollāsa deals exclusively with *Vaidyakīya Śāstra*. Physicians can find suitable directions here to diagnose properly the diseases with special reference to the *doṣas* involved before starting the course of treatment. Qualifications enumerated for a physician make an interesting study. Rāja Mānasollāsa quotes *Carakasaṁhitā* which prescribes the qualifications for a physician as under—

'Excellence in medical knowledge, an extensive practical experience, dexterity and purity are the essential qualities of a physician.'[38]

In the सूत्रस्थान of *Carakasaṁhitā,* there is a clear instruction for a physician as under—

'By virtue of his ability to bestow physical happiness and longevity, a physician is verily regarded as a donor of virtues, wealth and desired objects pertaining to this world and the world beyond.'[39]

The above analysis throws light on the nature of society during the period of Someśvara. Rāja Mānasollāsa assigns a unique place for a physician in society. In turn, the physician also rendered useful service to all the people.

श्रुते पर्यवदातत्वं बहुशो दृष्टकर्मता।
दाक्ष्यं शौचमिति ज्ञेयं वैद्ये गुणचतुष्टयम्।।

(चरकसंहिता सूत्रस्थान 9-6)

According to Caraka, excellence in knowledge can be had by attending on preceptors and studying scriptures. Purity in a physician helps the patient by dint of its spiritual force. Reputation as infallible in prescribing medicines is also one of the qualities of a physician and then he says about medicine.

Abundance, suitability, multiple form and potency, are the four qualities of medicament.[40]

There are patients who are averse to the taking of the juice of a drug, some others in paste *(kalka)* form. Similarly, there are certain diseases where a medicament is required to be administered in a particular form. For example, decoctions form a special therapy in the treatment of fever. So it is necessary that the medicaments are amenable to preparations according to various pharmaceutical processes. Moreover, medicaments should be potent and free from infections and dampness.

According to Rāja Mānasollāsa, medicine should be as follows :

पक्कमेवौषधं हन्ति दोषं कोष्ठसमाश्रितम्।
अपक्कं न गुणं किञ्चित् कुरुते तत् सुधारसम्।।

Effective medicine only will act against the pathology in the body. Otherwise, there will be no improvement in the health condition.

Caraka mentions four qualities in a patient. These are : Good memory, obedience, fearlessness and uninhibited expression.[41]

Even though fearlessness and good memory are regarded as qualities of a patient, (for fear, anxiety and such other mental stresses, aggravate the disease), still sometimes shock and loss of memory are prescribed as positive treatment for patients. For example, one of the treatments prescribed for a patient suffering from insanity is that he should be got terrified actually by a snake (shock therapy), of course, with its teeth taken out as a measure of safety. (Present day electric shock therapy administered on mental patients may be mentioned here.) In cases of fevers recurring at regular intervals, it is necessary to take measures to make him forget the occurrence of fevers.

Rāja Mānasollāsa then proceeds to describe the features of physicians—

शस्त्रशास्त्रविदोवैद्यानभ्यासनिपणानपि।
ऊहापोहविवेकज्ञान् सुधाहस्तान् प्रियंवदान्॥ (1.19.139)

Such Vaidyas (physicians and surgeons) have to be appointed who are professional experts in physiology and surgery, skillful in experiments (medicine) and possessing good judgement and having a curative touch and soft spoken nature.

In Āyurveda, great emphasis has been laid upon the selection of proper medical text for study. Students and teachers of medicine should be of special nature as may be conducive to the study and practice of medicine. Ceremonies for the initiation of the students to the medical profession were invariably performed.

Selection of the Medical Texts : A person desirous of adopting medical profession should, first of all, carefully select a suitable text on medicine, depending upon his competence to undertake light or serious type of work, his willingness for short term or long term results, his habitat and age. There are several such texts available for physicians. Only such texts having the following characteristic features are to be followed. Texts which are—

1. Patronised by great, illustrious and wise physicians, those texts which are great and popular and are followed by wise persons;
2. Pregnant with ideas and respected by reputed experts;
3. Conducive to the intellectual growth of disciples of all the three categories, viz., highly intelligent, moderately intelligent and less intelligent;
4. Free from defects of repetition, transmitted by seers and have well-knit aphorisms together with commentaries thereon in proper order;
5. Which have elegant ideas to convey;
6. Free from vulgar and difficult expressions and have clear and unambiguous expressions;
7. Which convey ideas in an orderly manner;
8. Which primarily deal with the determination of real objects;
9. Which are free from contradictions;
10. Where there is no confusion relating to contexts;
11. Which convey ideas quickly; and
12. Which are equipped with definitions of etiology, symptomatology and therapeutics and illustrations.

An Ideal Medical Teacher

An ideal preceptor is one who is well-grounded in scriptures, equipped with practical knowledge, wise, skillful, whose prescriptions are infallible, who is pious, who has all the necessary equipments for treatment, who is not deficient in respect of any of the sense organs, who is acquainted with human nature and the rationale of treatment, whose knowledge is not overshadowed by the knowledge of other scriptures, who is free from vanity, envy and anger, who is hard working, who is affectionately disposed towards his disciples and who is capable of expressing his view with clarity. A preceptor possessed of such qualities infuses medical knowledge into a good disciple as the seasonal cloud helps bringing about good crop in a fertile land.

One should approach such a preceptor and respect him like fire, god, king, father and master with all care. After having obtained the knowledge of the entire scripture, through his blessings, one should strive again and again for achieving depth in scriptures, clarity of expression, comprehension of the various concepts and power of oration.

An Ideal Medical Student

A person having the following qualities should be chosen as a medical student.

1. transquility; 2. generosity; 3. aversion to mean acts; 4. normal condition of eyes, face and nasal ridge; 5. thin, red and clear tongue; 6. absence of any morbidity in teeth, lips and voice; 7. perseverance; 8. freedom from vanity; 9. presence of intellect, power of reasoning and memory; 10. liberal mindedness; 11. birth in the family of a physician or the one having the disposition of a physician; 12. inquisitiveness for truth; 13. physical perfection; 14. unimpaired senses; 15. modesty and absence of ego; 16. ability to understand the real meaning of things; 17. absence of irritability; 18. absence of addictions; 19. good character, purity, conduct, love for study, enthusiasm and sympathetic disposition; 20. devotion to study; 21. uninterrupted taste for the theory and practice of the science; 22. absence of greed and laziness; 23. good-will for living beings; 24. obedience for all the instructions of the preceptor; and 25. devotion to the preceptor.

Initiation of Study : During a favourable *muhūrta* (a unit of time consisting of 48 minutes and named as Śiva, Bhujanga, etc.) and an auspicious *kṣaṇa* (a division of the day used in astrological science), when the moon is auspicious by virture of its conjuction with either of *Puṣya, Hastā, Srāvaṇa* or *Aśvayuk* constellation, on an auspicious day of the light fortnight of *uttarāyaṇa* (summer solstice) the disciple should come observing fast, after bath, wearing a saffron coloured cloth and with fragrant material in hand. He should also bring with him *samidha* (dry twigs used for offering oblation), fire, ghee, sandal wood paste, earthen jar filled with water, garlands, lamps, golds, ornaments of gold, silver, jewels, pearls, coral, silken garments, *paridhi* or sticks of *palāśa (Butea monosperma* Kuntze) of one cubit in lenght for being placed in the four sides of *homakuṇḍa* (a rectangularly dug fire place for offering oblations), *Kuśa (Desmostachya bipinnata* Stapf), fried paddy, *sarṣapa (Brassica nigra* Koch), *akṣata* (unbroken dehuskd rice), white loose flowers and garlands, prepared out of them, food articles which promote intellect and sweet scented pastes.

When the disciple comes with the preparations mentioned above, the physician should get constructed a *sthaṇḍila* (an elevated place of the shape of a square and of four cubits in size) in an even and pure place having slope towards the east or the north. The place should be smeared with cow dung, spread with *kuśa* grass and provided with good border on all the four sides. This place should then be decorated with sandal paste, earthen jar, water, silken garments, gold, ornaments of gold, silver, jewels, pearls, corals and food articles. After performing *homa,* the student should be intitiated in to study.

An Ideal Physician

In Āyurveda physicians are classified into three categories as follows :

1. Pseudo physicians; 2. Feigned physicians; and 3. Genuine physicians.

Those who come to be known as physicians simply by virtue of the exhibition of the physician's box containing certain drugs, medical books, by bluffing and posing as physicians belong to the first category. They are ignorant of the science of medicine. They are simply counterfeits.

Those who attribute their association to persons accomplished in wealth, fame and knowledge also come to be known as physicians, even though they are not so. Persons of this category are to be regarded as feigned physicians.

Those who are accomplished in the administration of therapies and have insight as well as knowledge of therapeutics, are endowed with infallible success and can bring out happiness belong to the category of genuine physicians.

Attributes of a good physician : Physicians who are born in noble families, well read, and have practical experience, who are skillful, pure, whose medicinal prescriptions and surgical operations are infallible, who are self-controlled, who have all equipments and are endowed with healthy sense organs, who are acquainted with natural manifestations and those who have presence of mind are the saviours of life and destroyers of diseases. Such physicians are well-acquainted with the anatomy and physiology of the entire body, creation and growth of the body and origin and evolution of the universe. They are free from doubts regarding the etiology, premonitory signs and symptoms, actual signs and symptoms as well as management of diseases which are easily curable, curable with difficulty, and incurable.

They are well-versed with the following :

1. Three principles of the science of life (viz., etiology, symptomatology and management of good and bad health);
2. Fundamental principles and their elaboration;
3. Three sources of drugs;

4. Thirty-five roots and fruits; four types of fat; five types of salt, eight types of wine, eight types of milk and six plants whose latex and bark are useful;
5. Various types of drugs used in five elimination therapies;
6. Twenty-two types of gruel;
7. Thirty-two types of powders and ointments;
8. Six hundred types of purgatives;
9. Five hundred types of decoction;
10. Factors responsible for the maintenance of positive health including diet, drug, regimen, residence, movement, sleep, rest, quantity, collyrium, inhalation, unction, washing, non-suppression of manifested urges, suppression of psychic urges, physical exercise and wholesomeness for examining the sense organs;
11. Knowledge of the four aspects of therapeutics having sixteen factors;
12. Determination of the nature of diseases;
13. Three pursuits of life;
14. Various actions of *vāyu;*
15. Four types of unctuous substances prepared according to twenty-four methods with drugs of various tastes, permutation and combination of which are of sixty-four types;
16. Various methods of preparation of drugs and therapies for fomentation and purgation;
17. Diseases of head, etc.;
18. Summary of diseases caused by permutation and combination of various *doṣas*;
19. Ailments like carbuncle and abscess;
20. Three types of oedema and other diseases having swelling in one or the other part of the body;

21. Forty-eight types of diseases;
22. One hundred forty-types of diseases of *nanātmaja* variety (diseases caused specifically by one *doṣa*);
23. Etiology, signs, symptoms and management of despisable individuals who are either very corpulent or emaciated;
24. Useful and harmful nature of sleep, sleeplessness and excessive sleep along with their etiology and management;
25. Six therapeutic measures like lightening therapy etc.;
26. Signs, symptoms and treatment of diseases due to over-nourishment; and under nourishment;
27. Diseases caused by the vitiation of blood, viz., intoxication, fainting and syncope alongwith their etilogy, signs and symptoms and treatment by medicines and regimen;
28. Rules of dietetics, food preparations which are wholesome and unwholesome by nature;
29. The diet and regimen which are foremost in nature amongst their group;
30. Forty types of alcoholic preparations;
31. Determination of *dravya* (matter), *guṇa* (quality), *karman* (action), primary and secondary tastes;
32. Various types of incompatible food ingredients;
33. Ingredients of food and drinks classified into twelve groups along with their properties;
34. Properties of post-prandial drinks;
35. Nine factors required to be examined for determining the properties of food;
36. Digestive and metabolic processes;
37. Good and ill effects of wholesome and unwholesome food;

38. Diseases caused by the vitiation of various tissue elements alongwith their treatment in brief.
39. Ten resorts of life.

They understand the eight sections of *Āyurveda* in their entirety along with the scope of the science. They have the power of grasping, retention and understanding of the text. They apply their knowledge so acquired for the treatment of diseases with a view to bringing the *dhātus* to their normal state after determining the stage of the disease, their own ability and the properties of the drugs employed. They are imbued with memory, intelligence theoretical and practical knowledge. They nurture cordial feelings exactly like the mother, father, brother and kin towards all creatures. Physicians having such qualities cure their diseases, and give life to patients.

Characteristics of pseudo and feigned physicians : According to Caraka pseudo and feigned physicians are those who move about from one street to another in search of livelihood in the garb of physicians. Once they hear about somebody's sickness, they would surround him and start enumerating their own qualities loudly so that the patient could listen to them. If the patient is already under treatment they try to find fault again and again with the attending physician. They win over the friends of the patient by pleasing manners, back-biting and flattering. They also propagate that they are interested in a nominal remuneration only. After they succeed in winning over patient, they look at him again and again skillfuly trying to cover their ignorance. If they are not able to alleviate the disease, they proclaim that the patient lacked in proper equipment, attendance and self-control. As soon as the patient dies, they run away to some other place in some other garb. In the congregation of ordinary men they proclaim their ability in self-contradicting tones. Like an impatient person they speak ill of the patience of courageous individuals. In the event of their coming across a congregation of the wise, they immediately leave the place from a distance. In case they happen to have the smattering knowledge of some therapeutic formulate, they will never hesitate in quoting them without caring for the relevance to the topic. They do not expect any questions from others nor do they like to pose any such questions to others. They get perturbed by the question as if attacked by death. Nobody knows anything about their preceptor, disciple, classmate or even their opponents.

Pseudo-physicians in the garb of doctors try to catch the patient as the bird-catchers their prey in the net. They are far away from the textual knowledge, practical experience, knowledge about the time of administering the therapy and its dosage. They are like the messengers of death on the earth; hence, they should not be entertained.

A qualified physician is he, who is well-acquainted with the principles of treatment, who is wise, is well-versed in classics and is prompt in action. The patient, who is administered proper emesis and purgation therapies by such a physician surely attains happiness. On the other hand, if a person who only claims to be a physician without having any grounding (in the science of medicine) administers these therapies, the patients would subject themselves to further complications because of the excessive or inadequate administration of this therapy.

Such of the actions as bringing about equilibrium of *dhātus,* constitute treatment of diseases. This, in fact, is the duty of the physician. The purpose of such action is to prevent the disturbance of the equilibrium of *dhātus* and maintain their equilibrium. By avoiding discrodant causing factors and adopting those responsible for the maintenance of equilibrium, discordance of *dhātus* is automatically prevented and their normal state of equilibrium is maintained. By taking recourse to concordant factors, the physician well-versed in treatment brings about equilibrium of *dhātus* and so he is the bestower of physical happiness and longevity. By virtue of his ability to bestow physical happiness and longevity, such a physician is verily regarded as a donor of virtue, wealth and desires pertaining to this world and the world beyond.

Examination of Patients

To ascertain the exact nature of the disease, the Āyurvedic physician, for the most part, depends upon eight types of examination of the patient before prescribing any medicine. These are the examination of (1) Pulse, (2) Urine, (3) Stool, (4) Tongue, (5) Voice, (6) Touch (skin), (7) Eyes, and (8) General physical features *(ākṛti)*. These examinations are conducted keeping in view the fundamental principles of Āyurveda. Thus, they are entirely different from the examination of pulse etc., by the modern medical doctors.

(1) *Pulse Examination* : It is carried out in the early morning when the patient's stomach is empty. It is prohibited immediately after bath, food and oil massage because the pulse then becomes erratic and does not indicate the correct condition of the patient. Similarly, a patient who is hungry and thirsty is not suitable for the purpose of pulse examination.

Pulse examination is carried out through the help of the radial artery. It is located in the place about half an inch below the wrist. In the case of males the pulse of right hand in the case of females that of the left hand is examined. For this purpose the arm should be stretched properly and the hand should be kept in slightly flexed position. Simultaneously, the fingers including the thumb should be in a stretched position. The physician should examine the pulse by the help of his right hand. Three fingers namely the index, the midle and the ring fingers are used for pulse examination. They are kept over the pulse, the index finger remaining near the thumb. Gentle and uniform pressure is applied through the tips of these fingers over the pulse and the pulsation of the artery is felt. The physician has to put pressure and release it repeatedly to correctly ascertain the exact finger on which the pulsation is felt more. If the pulsation is felt over the index finger *vāyu* is dominant in the patient.

Feeling in middle finger indicates the dominance of *pitta* and in ring finger indicates aggravation of *kapha* in the body of the patient.

Apart from this, the physician has also to ascertain the movement of the pulse. If the movement of the pulse is felt like the motion of a snake or a leech, it indicates the dominance of *vāyu.* If there is dominance of *pitta* then the pulse moves like a crow or a sparrow or a frog. In the case of *kapha* the movement of pulse is like that of a swan or a peacock or a cock. If the pulse at times moves like the snake and at some other time like a crow then there is dominance of *vāyu* and *kapha.* Movement of the pulse like a monkey and a swan indicates the dominance of *pitta* and *kapha.* When all the three *doṣas* are vitiated then the pulse moves like a wood-pecker bird.

If the pulse is regular, continuously for thirty times, then the patient is sure to survive. If there are interruptions, then this indicates imminent death. Apart from what has been stated above, in Āyurvedic texts, there is an elaborate description regarding the nature of the pulse in different diseases, and this is very frequently used by the physicians as the means to probe the diseases.

2. *Urine Examination* : For the examination of urine, it should be collected during the last quarter of the night. It should be stored in a glass container. The examination should, however, start after sunrise. The urine that comes out in the beginning should be discarded and the remaining urine should be collected for examination.

If there is dominance of *vāyu,* the urine becomes pale yellow in colour. If there is dominance of *kapha*, then the colour becomes white and there is a lot of foam in the urine. Yellow or red colour of the urine indicates the dominance of *pitta.*

In a clean wide-mouth glass container urine should be kept and over the surface of the urine, a few drops of oil should be dropped through a dropper. If the oil spreads immediately then the patient is curable and if the oil drops spread slowly, then the patient is difficult of cure. If the oil drops go down the urine then the patient is sure to die. If a patient suffers from indigestion, then his urine looks like fresh lime juice and sandalwood paste. If a patient is suffering from a disease caused by indigestion, his urine looks like the rice wash. If a patient suffers from acute fever, the urine becomes more in quantity and takes a cloudy colour.

If the oil drops spread towards the east then the patient is likely to get cured of his ailment very soon. Spreading of the oil drops towards south is indicative of a patient's suffering from fever which will slowly disappear. If they spread north or west, the patient undoubtedly is free from any disease. If the oil spreads towards south-east direction and holes appear in the oil, then the patient is sure to die. In Āyurvedic texts, there is an elaborate description about the diagnostic and prognostic value of urine examination.

3. *Stool Examination* : If there is dominance of *vāyu,* then the stool becomes hard and dry. Yellow colour of the stool indicates the aggravation of *pitta,* and white colour indicates predominance of *kapha.* When all the three *doṣas* are aggravated, then the stool carries three different colours. If *vāyu* is aggravated, then stool comes in pieces and it is rough, smoky and foamy.

If a small portion of the stool is dropped over water and it sinks, then it indicates the presence of *āma,* i.e., undigested or unmetabolised product in it. If it floats in water, then it indicates that stool is free from any such defect. Āyurvedic texts are replete with references to different colours, consistency, smell, etc., of the stool in different diseased conditions.

4. *Tongue* : When *vāyu* is aggravated, the tongue is cold and rough to touch and cracks appear in it. Predominance of *pitta* is indicated by the red or blue colour of the tongue. If *kapha* is predominant, then the tongue is white and exceedingly

slimy. When all the three *doṣas* are aggravated, then the tongue is black in colour and there are thorny eruptions over it.

5. *Voice* : If there is dominance of *kapha* then the voice becomes heavy. Clear and sharp voice indicates the dominance of *pitta.* Dry and hoarse voice is indicative of *vāyu* dominance.

6. *Touch* (skin) : The skin is hot if the patient is suffering from a disease caused by *pitta.* If the disease is caused by *vāta* then the skin is cold. The skin becomes moist and wet, if there is dominance of *kapha.*

7. *Eyes* : The eyes of a person suffering from diseases caused by *vāyu* are dry and smoky. The patient always gets burning sensation inside the eyes. If he suffers from a disease caused by *pitta* then there is aversion to light and burning sensation in eyes. The eyes become yellow in colour in such cases. Unctuousness and dullness of eyes indicate the predominance of *kapha*. The eyes of such patients are usually moist and there is profuse lachrymation. The conditions of the eyes are very significant to determine the prognosis of a disease.

8. *Physical Features* : Patients dominated by *vāyu* have mostly dry and cracked skin and hair. They do not like cold things and there is absence of patience, memory, intellect, effort and friendship in them. Such patients usually are talkative. Patients suffering from diseases caused by *pitta* are exceedingly thirsty and hungry. Their skin becomes yellow in colour and hot. The palm of the hand, the sole of the feet and face carry a coppery colour. They are usually aggressive and egoistic, having less of hair and the hair is slightly reddish in colour. The patient suffering from diseases caused by *kapha* have compact joints, bones and muscles. They do not suffer from excess of thirst, hunger, grief and pain.

Examination of Diseases : For proper treatment of a disease, it is essential to determine the exact nature of the disease with special reference to the *doṣas, dhātus, malas, srotas* and *agnis* involved in its manifestation. Some of these diseases are given names and for some others, names are not available. In fact Āyurvedic classics emphasise upon the physician not to be very particular about the name of the disease. According to these classics, names are attributed to some of these diseases only by way of example to facilitate the physician to ascertain and understand the gamut of remaining diseases for which names are not furnished. Since their number is very vast, it is not possible to name all of them. In respect of each disease whether named or unnamed, the following points need careful examination :

1. *Nidāna* or the cause of the disease;
2. *Pūrvarūpa* or the premonitory signs and symptoms;
3. *Rūpa* or the actual signs and symptoms of the disease;
4. *Upaśaya* or exploratory therapy; and
5. *Samprāpti* or the mode of manifestation of the disease.

The causes of all diseases have been classified in Āyurveda into the following three categories;

I. Intellectual blashphemy *(Prajñāparādha)*

II. Unwholesome conjunction of sense organs with their objects *(Asātmyendriyārtha saṁyoga)*

III. Vagaries of weather and time (*Kāla-pariṇāma)*

I. *Intellectual Blashphemy (Prajñāparādha)* : A person whose intellect, patience and memory are impaired, subjects himself to intellectual blashphemy by virtue of his bad action. This intellectual blashphemy aggravates all the *doṣas.*

Forcible stimulation of natural urges and suppression of the manifested ones, exhibition of undue strength, overin-dulgence in sexual act, negligence of the time of treatment, initiation of action in improper time (i.e., non-utilisation, excessive utilisation and wrong utilisation of therapies), loss of modesty and good conduct, disrespect for respectable ones, enjoyment of harmful objects, resorting to the factors which are responsible for the causation of madness, movements without any regard for temporal or local propriety, friendship with persons of bad actions, avoidance of the healthy activities, malice, vanity, fear, anger, greed, ignorance, intoxication and bewilderment or bad actions arising out of any of them or other physical evil acts arising out of *rajas* and *tamas* constitute intellectual blashphemy leading to the causation of various ailments.

II. *Unwholesome conjunction of sense organs with their objects* : This includes excessive utilisation, non-utilisation and wrong utilisation of objects, of senses, acts and time. For example, excessive gazing at the highly illuminous substance would constitute excessive utilisation of the visual organs. Not looking at anything at all would amount to its non-utilisation. Similarly, its wrong utilisation would be to see things too close or too far away, or things that are awful or terrifying, or are surprising, contemptuous, frightful, deformed and alarming.

Excessive utilisation of auditory objects would be to hear uproarious noise coming out of thunder and kettledrum, loud cries, etc. Its non-utilisation would be not to hear anything at all. Hearing of harsh words, news about the death of friends, assaulting, insulting and terrifying sounds constitute the wrong utilisation.

Smell of exceedingly sharp, acute and intoxication odours constitute an excessive utilisation of olfactory sense organ. Not to smell at all is its non-utilisation. Its wrong utilisation is the smell of exceedingly putrid, unpleasant, dirty, putrified and cadaverous odour and poisonous gas.

Similarly, excessive intake of various substances having various tastes, would amount to over-utilisation of gustatory sense faculty. Not to use it at all is its non-utilisation. The use of bath, massage and unction and other hot and cold substances without observing the prescribed order, touch of uneven place, dirty objects, bacteria and injurious touch constitute its wrong utilisation.

III. *Vagaries of weather and time* : A year is the unit of time which is further sub-divided into winter *(hemanta)*, summer *(grīṣma)* and rains *(varṣā)*, characterised by cold, heat and rainfall respectively. If a particular season manifests itself excessively, this should be regarded as excessive utilisation of time. If the season manifests itself in lesser measure, it would be its non-utilisation. If on the other hand, characteristics of a season are contrary to the normal ones, this would be wrong utilisation. If on the other hand, characteristics of a season are contrary to the normal ones, this would be wrong utilisation (for example, rainfall in winter, cold in the rainy season, etc.) A person exposed to these vagaries of seasons becomes a victim of many diseases.

According to Caraka, knowledge of the science of medicine is likened to the light for the purpose of illumination; one's own mental faculty to the eye (for the purpose of seeing things). A physician endowed with both of them, that is scriptural knowledge and his own intelligence, does not commit mistakes during the course of his treatment of a patient.

As the remaining three factors of treatment depend on the quality of the physician, a physician should always try to enrich his own qualities.[42]

Knowledge gained from the study of scriptures (*vaināyakī buddhi*) can be fully utilised only when a physician is endowed with good intelligence of his own.

मैत्री कारुण्यमार्तेषु शक्ये प्रीतिरुपेक्षणम्।
प्रकृतिस्थेषु भूतेषु वैद्यवृत्तिश्चतुर्विधा।।

(चरकसंहिता-सूत्रस्थान 9-26)

Physician should be sympathetic and kind to all patients, should be concerned with those who are likely to be cured and should feel detached with those are towards death. These are four disciplines for a physician.

Caraka says, "the curable diseases are cured by medicines possessing opposite qualities, (when) administered with due regard to the place, dose and time. No medicine is to be prescribed for incurable diseases.[43]

It is true that diseases are cured by drugs of opposite qualities. This is not all. It is necessary to take into account the place where the drugs are produced, the physical condition of the patient, the appropriate dose of the drug, the seasonal variation as well as the age of the patient. Unless all these are taken into account, simply the drugs of opposite qualities will not eradicate diseases. This justifies the ten-fold classification of the factors to be examined in connection with the cure of diseases, i.e., the *doṣas* affected, medicine, place, time, power of resistence in the body, conditions of the body, diet and its wholesomeness, mind, constitution of the body and age.

But even if all the above factors are taken into account, the drugs will have effect only on the diseases that are curable in nature. Certain diseases are incurable. For them, no medicine can be prescribed. It might be argued that there is no disease which cannot be cured by the sages, well-versed in the method of administration of elixirs, performance of penance, *japa* and *yoga*. Such wise persons can even overcome death. Thus, it might not be correct to say that no medicine can be prescribed for incurable diseases. But the statement in the above verse relates only to the physicians in general and not to the exceptional types of the sages, mentioned above.

The fact that a given disease is incurable can be determined by the symptoms indicative of approaching death (*ariṣṭa lakṣaṇa*). Such symptoms are of two types. Symptoms of the first category are bound to result in death and those of the second category may not result in death. Although, according to some, even such symptoms are indicative of the unavoidability of death. Thus, whenever, the symptoms indicative of approaching death occur, it is to be concluded that the patient must die, sooner or later. But even for such cases the use of elixirs, performance of penance, etc., are prescribed as efficacious therapies. Such therapies, however, are not accessible to a common man. So, for the purpose of the Āyurvedic prescriptions in general, the cases, where symptoms indicative of approaching death occur, are incurable in nature and as such, need not be treated at all.

Ap and *pṛthvī* constitute the substratum for the manifestation of taste *(rasa)* which is the object of gustatory sense organ (*rasanendriya*). As to the specific qualities of taste (*rasa*) three *pañcamahābhūtas (ākāśa vāyu* and *tejas)* are responsible for their manifestation.[44]

Rasa or taste is the object of gustatory sense organ, as distinct from the objects of the other sense organs. Primarily *ap* is the substratum of *rasa.* Besides, *pṛthvī* also indirectly serves as a substratum thereof.

The qualities of preceding basic elements (*ākāśa, vāyu, agni, ap* and *pṛthvī)* are included in the succeeding ones; so the qualities of *ap* are automatically included in *pṛthvī.* To sum up, *ap* and *pṛthvī* are the substrata for the manifestation of taste (*rasa).* That is to say, taste (*rasa*) can manifest itself only through *ap* and *pṛthvī.* These two *mahābhūtas,* (in addition to the remaining three) are also responsible for the manifestation of specific *rasas* like sweet, etc. For example, taste is sweet when there is predominance of the qualities of *ap* and it is sour when the qualities of *pṛthvī* and *tejas* are predominant.

The three basic elements, viz., *ākāśa, vāyu* and *tejas,* are only efficient causes of the manifestation of specific qualities of taste. By no means, they can be treated as substrata thereof. These three basic elements have their effects jointly and severally leading to their various degrees, like sweet, sweeter and the sweetest by the process of premutation and combination.

According to Rāja Mānasollāsa *kāla,* i.e., time, is also one of the factors for the manifestation of the various types and degrees of tastes. It says—

ज्ञात्वा निदानं व्याधीनां स्वरूपं लक्षणैः स्फुटम्।
देशकालानुसारेण सात्म्यंप्रकृतितत्त्वतः।। (1.19.144)

Appropriate treatment is to be provided to the patient in tune with the time and location, after learning about the pace of the disease and nature through its symptoms. *Āyurvedaśāstra* gives some information about treatment.

In the same way, we define good suggestions about various treatments.[45]

1. After a thorough study of '*Śāstras*', the great sages declared fourfold gifts for becoming happy here and hereafter. Fearlessness for the frightened, medicine for the sick, knowledge for the seeker of knowledge and food for the hungry are these four gifts.[46]
2. Life-saving treatment through medicine is equivalant to thousands of great sacrifices conducted for obtaining peace of mind.[47]
3. Just as the expanse of the sky is beyond the knowledge of gods, no one knows the limits of sanctity obtained by curing diseases.[48]
4. A healthy body is a means for attaining the four ultimate goals of life, Dharma, Artha, Kāma and Mokṣa—faith, wealth, enjoyment and liberation. A person free from sickness becomes eligible to enjoy the above fourfold gifts.[49]
5. Providing relief for a tired person, treatment of the sick, worship of gods, washing the feet of a guest and removal of remnants after their meal are equal to sacred duties.[50]

In fact, in spite of taste being directly related to *ap,* its manifestation necessarily requires the presence of *pṛthvī* in it. For taste cannot manifest itself without being related to *pṛthvī.*

According to *Caraka Saṁhitā*—drugs having sweet, sour and saline taste alleviate *vāta;* those having astringent, sweet and bitter (tastes) alleviate *pitta* and those having astringent, pungent and bitter (tastes) alleviate *kapha.*[51]

Vāta has in fact no taste. Even then the drugs having sweet, sour and saline tastes alleviate it. This is so because the tastes of the drugs possess their accessary qualities like unctuousness and as such are of opposite qualities. The various tastes can either alleviate or aggravate *doṣas*. Thus, these tastes which cannot alleviate, do necessarily aggravate the *doṣas*. For example, drugs of sweet, sour and saline tastes alleviate *vāta*. It automatically follows that those having astringent, bitter and pungent tastes would aggravate *vāta*. Similarly, *pitta* is aggravated by pungent, sour and saline drugs, and *kapha* by sweet, sour and saline drugs.

According to Caraka, only that, which can bring about a cure, is a correct medicine. It is only he who can relieve his patients of their ailments is the best physician.[52]

For the purpose of the science of medicine, it is necessary to explain the qualities of correct medicine and a good physician. It is only that which possesses the requisite curative values is to be treated as a correct medicine. As regards physician, he should first of all know the principles underlying the correct application of medicines. Unless he knows it, he will not be able to relieve his patients of their ailments. Even if perchance, medicines selected by him at random succeed in alleviating ailments, the credit is not his; it is just accidental. Thus, only he who can, by dint of his proficiency in the science, can select proper medicine and help cure diseases, can be regarded as the best physician.

As elsewhere, in the field of medicine also, the effect implies the existence of a cause. If a disease is cured, it naturally implies that proper therapy possessing the requisite curative properties has been administered, but for which, the disease could not have been cured. Similarly, if there is a success in the treatment of a disease, it also implies that the physician is proficient in the science of medicine.

We know already that diet or food for satisfying hunger is one of the biological needs of all the living beings in the world. To whatever category one may belong to, the plant, the animal and the human being, require food for growth and to sustain themselves. We will confine ourselves to the food of the human beings as advocated in Āyurveda not only for the growth but also to sustain the health. The principle is more to prevent diseases than to cure them. Three things are important in medical science, medicine (*auṣadha*), diet *(anna)* and activity *(vihāra)* to keep the normalcy of the body and mind, ultimately to bring comfort.

In Rāja Mānasollāsa, in *Annabhoga* chapter, we see the names of many famous articles of food and the directions as to the preparations of various dishes.

In modern science, food articles are primarily classified depending upon their chemical composition, namely, carbohydrate, protein, fat, vitamins, minerals, etc. In Āyurveda, such classification is based on the biological action of the food articles and their *rasa* (taste). For example, all varieties of rice may be treated as of one group on the basis of their carbohydrate content. But Āyurveda considers that freshly harvested rice is heavy for digestion. It aggravates *kapha.* If used continuously, it is considered to produce many complications. But old rice is useful for an average person. The freshly harvested rice produces more fat in the body than the old rice. Thus, for an emaciated individual having good digestive power, freshly harvested rice is nutritious, whereas for a fat person, even without good digestive power, old rice is nutritious.

Rāja Mānasollāsa says that rice is to be divided into eight varieties. i.e.,

रक्तशालिर्महाशालिर्गन्धशालिः कलिङ्गकाः ।
मुण्डशालिः शालिः सूक्ष्मशालिः सषष्ठिकः ।।

(3.13.1346)

Botanically all of them belong to the same genus and species. The botanical name is *Oryza sativa* Linn. But, according to Āyurveda, there is a great difference in their nutritive value.

There are many other types of food ingredients which chemically contain starch. But they are considered to produce a depletive effect on the human body. For example, *koradūṣa (Paspalum scrobiculatum)* type of corn produces depletive effect and reduces fat of the body expeditiously.

Pulses contain mostly protein. But, according to Āyurveda, some of them like *māṣa (Phascolus radiatus* Linn.) is heavy for digestion and it produces more fat in the body whereas *mudga (Phaseolus mungo* Linn.) is considered to be light for digestion and it reduces fat in the body. *Kulattha (Dolichos biflorus* Linn.), on the other hand, is exceedingly nutritious.

Āyurveda lays a great deal of emphasis upon proper diet for the treatment of patients. For each and every disease, wholesome and unwholesome food ingredients have been described.

Classification of Ingredients of Food and Drinks : In Āyurveda, ingredients used for food and drinks have been classified into 12 groups as below :

1. *Śūkadhānya* (corns with bristles) 2. *Samīdhānya* (pulses) 3. *Māṁsa* (Meat) 4. *Śāka* (vegetables) 5. *Phala* (fruits) 6. *Harita* (salads) 7. *Madya* (wines) 8. *Ambu* (water) 9. *Gorasa* (milk and milk products) 10. *Ikṣuvikāra* (products of sugar cane) 11. *Kṛtānna* (prepared food articles) 12. *Āhārayogin* (accessary food articles).

Āyurveda advocates both vegetarian and non-vegetarian diets not only for *svāstha* or healthy person, but also for unhealthy persons. There is a word in Āyurvedic literature which is *sātmīyatā* and that means the one for which the individual is acclamatised or used to, be it medicine or diet. The uncongenial food will not help the growth of a person. Moreover, diet of an individual depends on the availability of food in the region. And people in that region by experience find out what is wholesome and good for growth and what is injurious and prevents growth. By tradition and custom based on the experience of the forefathers, dietary regulations have been adopted by successive generations of people in that climatic condition and as the food is a question of survival of species in that region, the question of vegetarian and non-vegetarian does not count. In ancient India, the literature mentions that non-vegetarian food was served even by Ṛṣis and others. In medicine, as far as Āyurveda is concerned, there is no place either for sentimentality or emotional involvement. That is why the characteristics of every known animal food are described and the reaction caused by them when taken in both in health and ill-health are described. In *Aṣṭāṅga Hṛdaya* of Vāgbhaṭa, there is a chapter called *Anna svarūpavijñānīya,* the dietetics. In that chapter, the names, quality and characteristics of varieties of cereals (*śāli ṣaṣṭika),* millets—(*tṛṇa dhānya),* pulses (*śimbī dhānya*) are described. In the same way there is *māṁsa varga* or non-vegetarian diet in which eleven different kinds of non-vegetarian food items are described. And in each class, different animals, birds, reptiles and marine products are described. Even the flesh of carnivorous animals is advocated.

In Rāja Mānasollāsa while describing non-vegetarian preparations the method of removing the hair of a wild bear is given as follows :

पञ्चाङ्गपट्टवद्वेष्य वर्तिबद्धोज्ज्वलावपा।
अङ्गुलद्वयमानेन खण्डांस्तस्याः प्रकल्पयेत्।। (3.13.1499)

The animal should first be covered with a white piece of cloth. Boiling water should then be poured on the body of the boar with the help of a *Gandaka* (a vessel used for taking water from big earthen pot) with a handle slowly till the hair are so shaken from the roots that they can be easily removed by hands. The remainder may then be removed with the help of a pair of scissors. Another method of removing the hair from the body is to besmear it with mud and burn the skin with fire made of grass while treating of the preparation of खण्ड्स of वपा.

Some of the animals and birds could not be identified as the descriptions are so vast. Having described the characteristics of all the non-vegetarian and vegetarian food items, descriptions are also found, in Rāja Mānasollāsa as to which of the animals' or birds' flesh or marine product is good for health and in which seasons they have to be consumed.

Then, there is the description of vegetables *śākavarga,* where vegetables like brinjals, pumpkins, etc., and also various leafy vegetables are described. Their use in health and how they can be used in ill-health are explained.

Having classified the different articles which go as dietery articles, now the question is, how Āyurveda found the utility of them in various conditions. We know that in those ancient times, there were no laboratories to analyse and find out the contents in them or the technique of experiments concerned with animals. They were able to describe the qualities of the food and how the body utilises them to build up the various tissues of the body. They should have had a methodology. They classified the substances according to their tastes-*rasas*. They have said that for the growth of the body one is better than the other, in the reverse order. So the article with astringent taste makes a person shed weight and strength. Then the characteristic of the article is described from the standpoint of easy digestion.[53] They use the word *guṇa* for this. An article having *guruguṇa* takes longer time to get digested than that which is easily digested-*laghu. Anna* prepared of rice is quickly digested but *Anna* prepared from Sorghum (*rava* of jawar) takes longer time for digestion. This heavy (*guru)* and *(laghu)* light, should not be confused with its atomic weight but understood only from the standpoint of digestion.

The third point is *vīrya* or potency. There are only two activities in the body—one is anabolic (constructive) which builds up and another is ketabolic (destructive). The diet articles which possess *śīta vīrya,* are generally of anabolic nature i.e., they aid the growth of a person and the other *uṣṇa vīrya* mars the growth of an individual. All articles described come under these two categories. The fourth point is *vipāka.*[54] *Vipāka* means metabolism, *Viśeṣapāka.* A substance that is taken in, gets digested in the gastro-intestinal tract which is called *avasthā-pāka*— the different digestion that takes place from the mouth, stomach and small intestines. This is done by the *jaṭharāgni* or the various digestive fluids and enzymes that are secreted in the gastro-intestinal tract. There, when it becomes chyle and in Āyurvedic language *anna rasa,* it enters into the circulation to build up various tissues from blood to semen. This is done by the combined effort of the *bhūtāgni* and *dhātvagni.* In modern parlance, one can say that these are the biochemical changes brought on by the various enzymes. Āyurveda describes *sapta-dhātus*—seven elements namely, *rasa, rakta, māṁsa, medhas, asthi, majja* and *sūkta.* Each one of these tissues or *dhātus* has got digestive agents and from the digested food materials that is circulating in the body, the *dhātvagnis* or the digestive agents absorb and convert it to their needs. That is to say, from the food materials the blood takes its own materials which will replenish its wastage and the muscles will take what is needed, etc. Even before this happens, there are five *bhūtāgnis* which disintegrate the materials in the intestines and continue the process to the tissues also. So, if the diet article is taken, its metabolism or *dhātu pariṇāma* is done by 13 *agnis* or digestive agents. This is called *niṣṭa pāka*—the ultimate absorption of the food. We start with *avasthā pāka* in the gastro-intestinal tract and end with *niṣṭa pāka,* ultimate absorption of the food. If any one of these thirteen *agnis* is defective, then the food is not utilised for the growth and maintenance of the body.

Āyurveda plans the food requirement of a person not only after he is born, but also during the embryonic growth. *Suśrūta Saṁhitā,* describes the regimen for pregnant women, advising what food they should take and what should be their mental and emotional attitudes for the proper growth of the foetus. One peculiarity in this is that Suśrūta advocates different items of food from month to month depending perhaps on the growth of various organs and parts of the foetus. From the fourth month, the *garbhiṇī* or pregnant woman is called *dauhṛdī,* which means one who has two hearts, hers and that of the foetus. From that month onwards she has yearnings for various things. This is called *dauhṛdaṁ.* From the fifth month onwards the intelligence of the foetus develops and so more of milk and ghee in diet is advocated.

After delivery and during the period of lactation, to increase the breast milk, certain diets are given—garlic, fish, drumstick leaves and fruits, unfermented toddy, etc. The childhood is divided into three stages : *kṣīrāśi,* the child that depends on milk only and *kṣīra-annāśi* which depends on prepared food. And if mother's milk is not available or is insufficient, either cow's milk or goat's milk diluting it to suit the age of the child is given. Along with milk, if solid food is to be given, the grains are fried, powered, cooked and given (*saktu*).

One of the important contributions of Āyurvedic dietetics is recommendation of food according to the various seasons.[55] The year is divided into six seasons. According to the seasonal changes, the requirement of food differs and the variation in the quality of the food also changes. For example, in cold season and rainy season one should have more of the food articles which are sweet, sour and saltish; in *Vasanta,* pungent, astringent and bitter food; in summer, more of sweet things; in October-November—*Śaratkāla*—sweet and bitter and astringent food. In the same way, the fat content of the food also differs from season to season. The idea is that, *vāta, pitta* and *kapha,* the *doṣas* that maintain the body, get changed by the seasonal variation and to bring them to normalcy, the variation of the food becomes necessary.

During the middle period of one's life there is not much change in the diet. That is to say, from the age of twenty to fifty, one has to take whatever his requirement is, both for satisfaction and maintenance of health. For vegetarians milk of cow and ghee are particularly recommended. दुग्धावतान् घृतपक्वाश्च सितया च विमिश्रितान्। (3.13.1387). While describing the quality of milk, it is mentioned that it prolongs life and wards off symptoms of senility. In describing the quality of ghee, it is mentioned that it increases the memory power, intelligence, strength of the body, longevity of life and strengthens the eye-sight. शस्तं धीस्मृतिमेधायुर्बलायुःशुक्रचक्षुषाम् (अष्टङ्ग०हृ०). It is said that if properly used milk can do good to the body. Buttermilk is reommended more than the curds. चूषेत मज्जिकां पश्चाद्दधि चाद्याऽत्ततो धनम्। (3.13. 1596). Even if curd is taken, it should be taken with honey, green gram, soup, etc. And two important vegetables that are recommended for every day use are *Harītaki* and *Āmalakī*. *(Terminalia Chebula* and *Emblica officinalis*). Both of them are good for digestion, increase intelligence and memory power and ward off symptoms of old age. Both of them can be used in raw form or in dry form. It is better to use *Āmalaki* in raw form and *Harītaki* in dry form.

Whatever may be the quality of the food items recommended in the Rāja Mānasollāsa, their use depends largely on tradition and custom. Apart from the economic condition of the people who use the food, social approval also is necessary. A man consists not only of the body but also of the mind and soul. These are the tripods on which man exists. So the intention of the dietery programme is to build the body without disturbing the qualities of the mind. We need not consider the soul for the present. The food one takes in, is capable of influencing the mind also.

Rāja Mānasollāsa advises to sip water everyday during meals. This, the author thinks, adds taste to the food and helps digestion. Someśvara's rule regarding the drinking of water is rather peculiar. He recommends that whenever the king is thirsty, he should drink water and should never think of time and circumstances, that is to say, whether it is morning of mid-night or whether he is with a full or an empty stomach. In this respect King Someśvara recommends that the rules of medical science may be violated.[56]

Therefore, food is divided under *sātvic, rājasic* and *tāmasic* food. *Satva, rajas* and *tamas* are the qualities of the mind and *vāta, pitta* and *kapha* are the qualities of the body. The choice of food articles should be according to the avocations of the person. It is to be decided whether one chooses non-competitive avocation or competitive profession. For the former one should use *sāttvic* food and for the latter preference is for *rājasic* food.

The *Taittiriya Upaniṣad* (II. 2) has aptly emphasised the importance of food. Everything that rests on this earth, moveable or immovable, is produced from food. Then they live by food. Food is the eldest born among the beings. Therefore, it is the medicament for all, for normal maintenance of physical and mental health and also for restoration of health after diseases.

Someśvara had mastered all the branches of worldly knowledge. His Sanskrit language is natural, simple, chaste and refined. His thoughts and ideas are so profound that they make one infer that he must have had liberal education in a systematic manner. It has been already shown how it is evident from the study of his Rāja Mānasollāsa that he had mastered thoroughly all the scriptures and the works in different branches of knowledge in Sanskrit.

Rāja Mānasollāsa is written for the sake of प्रजारञ्जन. According to Someśvara, just as the moon gives pleasure to the mankind by her light, this work does so by the rich knowledge embodied in it. Hence, he has very rightly said that the kings must study Rāja Mānasollāsa in the interest of the welfare of their subjects. He also suggests that scholars also should study this work for the development of their knowledge.

पुण्यौधानामपि च्र महतां वृद्धये बुद्धये च।। (1.20.308)

References

1. वसन्ते कटु चाश्नीयात्ग्रीष्मे मधुरशीतलम्।
वर्षासु च तथा क्षारं मधुरं शरदि स्मृतम्।।
हेमन्ते स्निग्धमुष्णं च शिशिरेऽप्युष्णमम्लकम्।
एवं भुञ्जीत यद्भूपो अन्तभोगः स कथ्यते।। (3.13.1599-1600)
2. विपरीतगुणस्तेषां स्वस्थवृत्तेर्विधिर्हितः।
समसर्वरसं सात्म्यं समधातोः प्रशस्यते।। (चरकसंहिता-सूत्रस्थान 41)
3. रसनार्थो रसस्तस्य द्रव्यमापः क्षितिस्तथा।
निर्वृत्तौ च विशेषे च प्रत्ययाः स्वादयस्त्रयः।। (चरकसंहिता-सूत्रस्थान 1.62)
4. जन्म तु द्रव्यरसयोरन्योन्यापेक्षिकं स्मृतम्।
अन्योन्यापेक्षिकं जन्म यथास्याद्देहदेहिनोः।। (सुश्रूतसंहिता-सू० 26.37)
5. पाको नास्ति विना वीर्यात् वीर्यं नास्ति विना रसात्। (चरकसंहिता-सूत्रस्थान 1.64)
6. असत्यवर्जनं कार्यं परद्रोहस्यवर्जनम्।
वर्जनं चाप्यगम्यानामभक्षस्य च वर्जनम्।। (1.1-14-308 एण्ड 2.19.1005-1030)
7. प्रकृतिकरणसंयोगाः राशिर्देशो विशिष्टकालश्च।
भोक्ता भोजननियमश्चेत्यष्टौ ज्ञेयभावाः स्युः।।
(षोडशाङ्गहृदयम्-स्वस्थवृत्तम्— Quoted in Dr. P. V. Sharma's p. 256, 58.)
8. मात्राशी स्यात्। आहारमात्रा पुनरग्निबलापेक्षिणी।। (चरकसंहिता-सूत्रस्थान 3)
9. cf. यावद्ध्यस्याशनमशितमनुपहत्य प्रकृतिं यथाकालं जरां गच्छति तावद्स्य मात्राप्रमाणं वेदितव्यं भवति।। (चरकसंहिता-सूत्रस्थान 4)
10. धर्मार्थकाममोक्षाणामारोग्यं मूलमुत्तमम्।।
रोगास्तस्यापहर्तारः श्रेयसो जीवितस्य च।
प्रादुर्भूतो मनुष्याणामन्तरायो महानयम्।।
कः स्यात्तेषांशमोपाय इत्युक्त्वा ध्यानमास्थिताः।
अथ ते शरणं शक्रं ददृशुर्ध्यानचक्षुषा।।
स वक्ष्यति शमोपायं यथावद्मरप्रभुः। (चरकसंहिता-सूत्रस्थान 1.15-17)
11. पूर्वभुक्तेऽजीर्णे पुनरशनं ज्ञेयमहितमध्यशनम्।
विषमाशनन्तु विषमं मात्राकलादिभिः प्रोक्तम्।।
समशनमिह तत् प्रोक्तं पथ्यापथ्यस्य यत्र साङ्कर्यम्।
विविधो मिथ्याहारस्त्वेषु नरैः सर्वथा त्याज्यः।।
(Quoted in P.V. Sharma's षोडशाङ्गहृदय-स्वस्थवृत्तम् 61-62, पृ० 256.)
12. द्वौ भागावन्तेन द्रवतस्त्वेकं प्रपूरयेज्जठरे।
रिक्तस्त्वेकः स्थाप्यः दोषाणां सम्यगयनाय।। *Ibid.*, 64.
13. Adelle Dairs—'Let's cook it right' (George Allen & Union Ltld., London 1971, p. 13) Quoted in M.N. Joshi's "Treatment of Secular Arts & Sciences in Someśvara's Rāja Mānasollāsa" Ph.D. Thesis (unpublished), K.U.D., p. 335.

14. *Ibid.*, pp. 363-364.
15. वसन्ते कटु चाश्नीयात् ग्रीष्मे मधुरशीतलम्।
    वर्षासु च तथा क्षारं मधुरं शरदि स्मृतम्।।
    हेमन्ते स्निग्धमुष्णं च शिशिरेऽप्युष्णमम्लकम्।
    एवं भुञ्जीत यद्रूपो अन्नभोगः स कथ्यते।। (3.14.1599-1600)
16. Quoted in आयुर्वेदोपदेशसंग्रहः आरोग्यसुभाषितानि By Dr. M.N. Joshi, p. 43.
17. अग्निस्तु पाककर्मण्यविनाभावेन साधको ज्ञेयः।
    ते संख्या त्रयोदश जाठर-भूतस्थ-धातुसंस्थाश्च।।
    तेषां सर्वाध्यक्षः ख्यातो वैश्वानरोऽनलो जठरे।
    यो हि चतुर्विधभुक्तं पचति रसार्थं मलार्थञ्च।।
    भूताग्नयस्तु पञ्च प्रत्येकं भुक्तनीतभूतांशम्।
    परिणमयन्ति यथास्वं भूतानां पोषणार्थं हि।।
    धात्वग्नयस्तु सप्त प्रत्येकं धातुमञ्जसाश्रित्य।
    भागत्रये पचन्ति स्थूले सूक्ष्मेऽतिसूक्ष्मे च।।
    स्थूलो भागः किट्टं सूक्ष्मः स्वो धातुभाग एव स्यात्।
    परिणम्यतेऽतिसूक्ष्मश्चोत्ताधातौ क्रमश्चैष:।।
    एवं पाकविधानात् परिणामो दृश्यते तनौ द्विविधः।
    एकः प्रसारभूतः किट्टाख्यस्त्याज्य एवान्यः।।
    अंतर्मुखः प्रसादः किट्टाख्योऽशोबहिर्मुखो विदितः।
    आद्यः प्रीणाति वपुः कुरुते मलिनं द्वितीयस्तु।
    (षोडशाङ्गहृदयम्-मौलिकसिद्धान्त: Dr. P.V. Sharma, p. 177)
18. All these (1-7) statements are quoted from—Āyurvedāchārya Bhāskar Govind Ghāṇekar's "*Vaidyakīya Subhāṣita Sāhityam*", Chaukhamba Sanskrit Samsthana, Varanasi, 1977.
19. सुजीर्णमन्नं, सुविचक्षणः सुतः
    सुशासिता स्त्री, नृपतिः सुसेवितः।
    सुचिन्त्य चोक्तं, सुविचार्य यत्कृतं
    सुदीर्घकालेऽपि न याति विक्रियाम्।। (हितोपदेश)
20. जीर्णभोजिनं व्याधिर्नोपसर्पति।। (चाणक्यसूत्र)
21. विद्याघातो ह्यनभ्यासः, स्त्रीणां घातः कुचैलता।
    व्याधीनां भोजनं जीर्णं, शत्रोर्घातः प्रपञ्चता।। (बृहस्पति)
22. दोषभीतेरनारम्भस्तत्कापुरुषलक्षणम्।
    कैरजीर्णभयाद्भ्रातर्भोजनं परिहीयते।। (हितोपदेश)
23. प्रायेणाहारवैषम्यादजीर्णं जायते नुणाम्।
    तन्मूलो रोगसङ्घातस्तद्विनाशाद्विनश्यति।। (अष्टाङ्गसंग्रह)
24. दुरधीता विषं विद्या, अजीर्णे भोजनं विषम्।
    विषं गोष्ठी दरिद्रस्य, वृद्धस्य तरुणी विषम्।। (चाणक्यशतक)

25. पथ्यमप्यमथ्याजीर्णे नाश्नीयात्।। (चाणक्यसूत्र)
26. सामादीनां प्रयोक्तारमशक्तं मन्वते द्विषः।
तस्माद् दण्डं प्रयुंजीत दण्डो हि वशकृन्नृणाम्। (2.20.1032)
तण्डनीतिर्यदा सम्यङ्नेतारमधितिष्ठति।
तदा विद्याविदः शेषा विद्याः सम्यगुपासते।।
त्रिवर्णोऽयं धर्ममूलो नरेन्द्र राज्यं चेदं धर्ममूलं वदन्ति।
धर्मे राजन्वर्तमानः स्वशक्त्या पुत्रान्सर्वान्पाहि कुन्तीसुतांश्च।
(कामन्दकीय नीतिसार, द्वितीय सर्ग महाभारत, आरण्यक पर्व 5.4)
27. क्षुद्ध्या सुप्रतिपन्नेषु कुर्यात्साधुपरिग्रहम्।
विग्रहं चाप्यशिष्टेषु निर्मर्यादेषु कारयेत्।। (महाभारत, आरण्यक पर्व। 49-48)
28. नियुक्तहस्तार्पितराज्यभारास्तिष्ठन्ति ये स्वैरविहारसाराः।
बिडालवृन्दाहितरुग्धमुद्राः स्वपन्ति ते मूढधियः क्षितीन्द्राः।।
ज्ञायेत मार्गः सलिलेतिमीनां पतत्रिणां व्योम्नि कदाचिदेषः।
अध्यक्षसिद्धेऽपि कृतावलोपा न ज्ञायतेऽमात्यजनस्य वृत्तिः। (यशस्तिलक 3-23-24)
29. दूतं चैव प्रकुर्वीत सर्वशास्त्रविशारदम्।
इंगितावारचेष्टज्ञं शुचिं दक्षम् कुलोद्गतम्।।
अनुरक्तः शुचिर्दक्षः स्मृतिमान् देशकालवित्।
वपुष्मान् नीतिभीर्वाग्मी दूतो राज्ञां प्रशस्यते।। (मनुस्मृति 6.63.64)
30. संध्याम्चोपास्य श्रुणुयादन्तर्वेश्मनि शास्त्रभृत्।
रहस्याख्यायिनाम् चैव प्रणिधीनाम् च चेष्टितम्।। (मनुस्मृति 7.22.3)
31. अदोषान् दूषयन् राजा दोषयुक्तानदण्डयन्।
अकीर्ति महतीमेति दुर्गतिं चाधिगच्छति।। (2.20.1244)
32. देशनाशश्च शत्रूणां जनांगच्छेदकस्तथा।
गोग्रहो धान्यहरणो बन्दिग्राहस्तथाऽपरः।।
देशहारो धनादानः सर्वस्वहराणोऽपरः।
दुर्गभङ्गः स्थानदाहो देशनिर्वासिकस्तथा।।
युद्धावहो महादण्डः शत्रुसंहारकारकः।
उपायानां तुरीयश्च कथितः सोमभूभुजा। (2.20-1035-1037)
33. देशधर्मान् जातिधर्मान् कुलधर्मांश्च शाश्वतान्।
पाषण्डगणधर्मांश्च शास्त्रेऽस्मिन्नुक्तवान् मनुः।। (मनुस्मृति 1.118)
34. अन्येषामपि देवानाम् निन्दां द्वेषं च वर्जयेत्।
देवं देवकुलं दृष्ट्वा नमस्कुर्यात्र लङ्घयेत्।
एवं च आस्तिकं भावमाश्रितः समतां गतः।
सर्वदेवप्रसादेन लभते सम्पदं वराम्।। (1.12.105-106)
35. पुत्राणामुपभोगोऽयमद्यः संपरिकीर्त्यते।
ऋतुकालमनुल्लङ्घ्य पुत्रार्थी सङ्गमाचरेत्।। (3-12-1245)
तृतीयो मासि संप्राप्ते कुर्यात्पुंसवनं नृपः। (3-12-1250)

एक द्विवत्सरस्यान्ते कारयेत् कर्णवेधनम्। (3-12-1278)
वत्सरद्वितीयादूर्ध्वं चूडाकार्या यथाकुलम्।। (3-12-1280)
शस्तेवारे शुभे लग्वे तिथौ च शुभशंसिनि।
अन्नप्राशनधिष्ण्येषु ध्रुवनक्षत्रवर्जिते।। (3-12-1282)
भौमे सौम्ये गुरौ शुक्रे कुर्यान्मौंजीनिबंधनम्।
वर्षे गर्भाष्टमे वाऽपि गर्भैकादशकेऽपि वा।। (3-12-1282-1283)
सम्प्राप्तयौवनान् पुत्रान् कृतगोदानमङ्गलान्।। 3-12-1305)
कुर्याद्विवाहं भूपालः पुत्रस्यामित्रकर्शिनः।
शोभने सुविशाले च मध्ये वेदिविराजिते।। (3-12-1309)

36. G.S. Dikshit—*Local self-Government in Mediaeval Karnataka*, Karnatak University, Dharwad,1964, p. 97.
37. परं पारंगताः सम्यगष्टङ्गे तु चिकित्सिते।
शस्त्रकर्मकलादक्षा मन्त्रे तन्त्रे च कोविदाः।। (2.2.139)
38. शस्त्रशास्त्रविदो वैद्यानभ्यासनिपुणानपि।
ऊहापोह विवेकज्ञान् सुधाहस्तान् प्रियंवदान्।।
अर्पयित्वा विचित्राणि भेषजानि पृथक् पृथक्।
निरालस्यांश्च धर्मज्ञान् प्रकल्प परिचारकान्।। (1.19.139-140)
39. धर्मस्यार्थस्यस कामस्य नृलोकस्योभयस्य च।
दाता संपद्यते वैद्यो दानाद् देहसुखायुषाम्।। (चरकसंहिता-सूत्रस्थान 16.38)
40. बहुता तत्रयोग्यत्वमनेकविधकल्पना।
संपच्चेति चतुष्कोऽयं द्रव्याणां गुण उच्यते।। (चरकसंहिता-सूत्रस्थान 9-7)
41. स्मृतिर्निर्देशकारित्वमभीरुत्वमथापि च।
ज्ञापकत्वं च रोगाणामातुरस्य गुणाः स्मृताः।। (चरकसंहिता-सूत्रस्थान 9-9)
42. शास्त्रं ज्योतिः प्रकाशार्थं दर्शनं बुद्धिरात्मनः।
ताभ्यां भिषक् सुयुक्ताभ्यां चिकित्सन्नापराध्यति।
चिकित्सते त्रयः पादा यस्माद्वैद्यव्यपाश्रयः।
तस्मात् प्रयत्नमातिष्टेद्भिषक् स्वगुणसंपदि।। (चरकसंहिता-सूत्रस्थान 9.24-25)
43. विपरीतगुणैर्देशमात्राकालोपपादितैः।
भेषजैर्विनिवर्तन्ते विकाराः साध्यसंमताः।।
साधनं न त्वसाध्यीनामुपदिश्यते। (चरकसंहिता-सूत्रस्थान 1.62)
44. रसनार्थो रसस्तस्य द्रव्यमापः क्षितिस्तथा।
निर्वृत्तौ च विशेषे च प्रत्ययाः खादयस्त्रयः।। (चरकसंहिता-सूत्रस्थान 1.64)
45. All these (1-5) statements are quoted from—Āyurvedāchārya Bhaskar Govind Ghāṇekar's *"Vaidyakīya Subhāṣita Sāhityam"*, Chaukhamba Sanskrit Samsthana, Varanasi, 1977.
46. इह चत्वारि दानानि प्रोक्तानि परमर्षिभिः।
विचार्य नानाशास्त्राणि शर्मणेऽत्र परत्र च।।

भीतेभ्यश्चाभयं देयं, व्याधितेभ्यस्तथौषधम्।
देया विद्यार्थिने विद्या, देयमन्नं क्षुधातुरे।। (काशीखण्ड)

47. एकतः क्रतवः सर्वे सहस्रवरदक्षिणाः।
अन्यतो रोगभीतानां प्राणिनां प्राणरक्षणम्।। (महाभारत)

48. आकाशस्य यथा नान्तः सुरैरप्यवगम्यते।
तद्वदारोग्यदानस्य नान्तो वै विद्यते क्वचित्।। (स्कन्दपुराण)

49. धर्मार्थकाममोक्षाणामारोग्यं साधनं यतः स्याच्चतुष्टयम्।
तस्मादारोग्य दानेन दद्दतं स्याच्चतुष्ट यम्।। (स्कन्दपुराण)

50. श्रान्तसंवाहनं रोगिपरिचर्या सुरार्चनम्।
पादशौचं द्विजोच्छिष्टमार्जनं गोप्रदानवत्।। (याज्ञवल्क्यस्मृति)

51. स्वाद्वम्ललवणा वायुं, कषायस्वादुतिक्तकाः।
जयन्ति पित्तं, श्लेष्माणं कषायकटुतिक्तकाः।। (चरकसंहिता-सूत्रस्थान 1-66)

52. तदेव युक्तं भैषज्यं यदारोग्याय कल्पते।
स चैव भिषजां श्रेष्ठो रोगेभ्यो यः प्रमोचयेत्।। (चरकसंहिता-सूत्रस्थान 1-134)

53. गुरूणाम् अर्धसौहित्यं लघूनां नातितृप्तता।। (अष्टाङ्ग हृदयम्, 1.8.2)

54. जाठरेणाग्निना योगाद्यदुदेति रसान्तरम्।
रसानां परिणामान्ते स विपाक इति स्मृतः।। (अ.हृ. 1.9.20)

55. शीते वर्षासु चाद्यांस्त्रीन् वसन्तेऽन्त्यान् रसान्भजेत्।
स्वादुं निदाघे शरदि स्वादुतिक्तकषायकान्।।
शरद्वसन्तयो रूक्षं शीतं घर्मघनान्तयोः।
अन्नपानं समासेन विपरीतमतोऽन्यदा।
नित्यं सर्वरसाभ्यासः स्वस्वाधिक्यमृतावृतौ।। (अ.हृ. 1.3.46-47)

56. पिपासां च जातायां स्वेच्छया पीयते जलम्।
नियमो नात्र कालस्य तृषावेगो न धार्यते।। (3.14.1603)

cf : पिबेद्घटसहस्रं तु यावन्नास्तमितो रविः।
अस्तङ्गते दिवानाथे बिन्दुरेको घटपते।।

Mānasollāsa, Gaekwad's Oriental Series No. 84, Int. p. 23.

Appendix

Glossary of Select Sanskrit Words

1. अष्टांग—Eight parts of Āyurveda—

   शल्य—Surgery.

   शालाक्य—Treatment of the diseases of Eye, Ear, Nose and Throat.

   कायचिकित्सा—The art of Healing.

   भूतविद्या—Treatment of diseases of super natural origin, with the use of medicines and natural powers (Demonology)

   कौमारभृत्य—Midwifery and care of children.

   रसायन तन्त्र—Promotion of health and longevity. (Toulogy).

   वाजीकरण तन्त्र—The science of developing sexual power and fecundity.

   अगद तन्त्र—Toxicology.

2. अग्रहार:—Royal gift of land to *Brāhmaṇas.*
3. अन्नाद—($\surd$अद्-to eat) eaten. eating food [eating the most].
4. अम्बु—Water Naigh. A kind of Andropogon.
5. अध्यशन—Eating too soon after a meal. (before the last meal is digested).
6. अपरा विद्या—The knowledge of science and ethics.
7. अभिमान—High opinion about one's self or self-conceit.

8. अवतारवाद—The theory of divine incarnation.
9. अहंकार—Egotism, Selfish, Self-consciousness or individualization.
10. आगम—The literature elucidating the different subjects of Vedas. Consideration of material powers. Tantra Śāstra.
11. आचार्यः—A preceptor, a master, or a learner, with practical knowledge. Knowing or teaching the rules, a spiritual guide or teacher especially one who invests the student with the sacrificial thread, and instructs him in the Vedas, in the law of sacrifice and religious mysteries.
12. आर्यावर्तः—Abode of the noble or excellent ones. The sacred land of the Āryans.
13. आस्तिक—A believer in God or a theist, antonym of non-believer or atheist.
14. आयुर्वेद—Scinece of life with all its aspects.
15. आहार— Food; eatables.
16. औषधि—A drug which removes a disease without impelling the other.
17. औषधि संरक्षिका—Female supervisors of a dispensary.
18. औपनिषदिकवर्ग—Teachers of religious and spiritual success.
19. इहलोक—'Aryāvarta' was said to be 'इहलोक' while the state of 'Svarga' was 'परलोक'.

    उत्तरे हिमवत्पार्श्वे पुण्ये सर्वगुणान्विते।

    पुण्यः क्षेम्यश्चकाम्यश्च स परोलोक उच्यते।।

    (महाभारत, शान्ति पर्व, अ० 8)

20. उपरस—Metal and minerals when used for medical purpose.
21. उपाध्यायः—A teacher; preceptor-who subsists by teaching a part of the Veda or Vedangas.

22. उत्साही—Powerful or mighty person. (उद्+√सह) to endure.
23. उद्भिद—Vegetable Kingdom.
24. ऋतुचर्या—Routine for seasons (रात्रिचर्या—Routine for night).
25. ऋषि:—Seers, who achieved the stage of *Dhāraṇa* (धारणा) in Yoga. They are given the ruling powers in *Narak.*
26. ऋत:—A scientific truth.
27. ऋक्—The name of the first Veda, ऋग्वेद (Ṛg-Veda) out of four Vedas यजु, साम and अथर्व.
28. ऋण:—Duties of individual for mother, father and teacher (Pitru, Ṛsis).
29. कर्मभोगवाद:—The *karma* theory, according to which one cannot escape the consequences of his deeds done in the present and past lives.
30. कला—An element of beauty or the science of beauty. (64 Kalas).
31. काय—(√ci, Pan. iii, 3-41). The body.
32. कुल—Family or race. Community.
33. कृतान्न—Food preparations. Or one who makes a meal.
34. क्षीरप—Drinking milk only.
35. क्षीरान्नद—Drinking milk and eating.
36. क्षय—To be diminished, food decrease.
37. क्षुधा—Hunger, to feel hungry.
38. गन्धार—The biggest province of *Svarga,* situated to the west of Panjāb or Kekaya Desh or that of the Sindhu river. *Gandharvas* stood first to rebel against the republic of *Svarga.* Afterwards Gandhar was rendered to be a province of Āryāvarta. *Gandharvas* developed highly in arts.
39. गुरुकुल:—The house of a Guru. Residence in the house of a Guru a pupil's life.

40. गुरु—Heavy, weighty (Heavy in the stomach-difficult to digest.)
41. गोष्ठी:—Meeting, assembly.
42. गोरस—Milk and Milk products.
43. चतुर्वर्ग:—Four aims of life, as

    1. धर्म: 2. अर्थ: 3. काम: 4. मोक्ष:
44. चय:—The accumulation of *Doṣas* according to seasons. there are three stages of it.

    1. चय 2. प्रकोप 3. प्रशम
45. चिकित्सा—Treatment; behaviour; manner of applying remedies. A process to achieve the health.
46. चिकित्सक:—One who cures a disease.
47. चैत्यपूजा—The worship of monuments.
48. छाया—The glare of the face. छाया दूरात्प्रकाशते (चरक)
49. जनपदोध्वंसी रोग—Epidemics.
50. जंगम—Animal kingdom.
51. जठराग्नि—Digestive stomach-fire.
52. जाति—Caste.
53. जीव—Soul, life, a person, immortal spirit of man.
54. तन्त्र:—Divination of actions. Doctrine; scientific work; principal part; Theory.
55. तमस्—Of heaviness; ignorance; anger, pride; sorrow. One of the three guṇas (सत्व; रजस्; and तमस्)
56. देह—The body ($\sqrt{}$dih-to mould).
57. दूत—An envoy.
58. दिनचर्या—Routine for day or the Regimen during day-time.
59. देश—Local habitation.

60. देहसिद्धि—Corporal divination.
61. देवनदी—They are four—

 1. Saraswati 2. Drishadwati

 3. Ganga 4. Yamuna

 Between these rivers *Devas* made a colony named *'Brahmāvarta'*. Manu mentions it as देव निर्मितं देशम् ब्रह्मावर्त्तम्. Sage Atri was living there.
62. धर्म—Duty, Rightousness or natural properties of a thing.
63. धन्व—A Desert, During the time of Āryāvarta, denoted the famous desert of Assyria.
64. धातु—The equivalent in English for धातु can be either Tissues, or Entities.
65. धात्री वर्ग—Wet nurses.
66. धातुशास्त्र—A description of metals to aid the medical science.
67. ध्वनि चिकित्सा—Treatment by sound.
68. नास्तिक—Atheist, Blasphemer. One who denies the existence of God.
69. नाड़ी विज्ञान—The scinece of examining pulse.
70. नीरजा—Leeches, blood sucking worm.
71. निरिन्द्रिय—Inorganic substances.
72. निदान—Etiology. Study of the cause of diseases.
73. निगम—Vedas or thorough knowledge.
74. परंपरा—Continuation, tradition.
75. परलोक—The state of *Svarga* flourishing on the Himālayas. It was strictly restricted for un-permitted persons, who lived in *Naraka*.

 उत्तरे हिमवत्पार्श्वे पुण्ये सर्वगुणान्विते। पुण्यः क्षेम्यश्चकाम्यश्च स परोलोक उच्यते।। इहस्थास्तत्र जायन्ते ये वै पुण्य कृतोजनाः।

 (महाभा०, शान्ति०, अ० 8,514,518)

76. पञ्चमहाभूता:—*Pṛthvi, Jala, Tejas, Vāyu* and *Ākāśa* are the five basic elements of the world.

77. पञ्चजन—Five sections of Āryans in Svarga :

 1. Devas. 2. Nagas.
 3. Yakṣas. 4. Gandharvas. 5. Kinnaras

78. परिसर—Environs.

79. पर्यावरण—Environment; Surrounding, covering.

80. पराविद्या:—Spiritual Knowledge.

81. परिचारिका—Midwives and Nurses.

82. परिनिर्वाण:—Redemption for ever.

83. पशुचिकित्सा—Veterinary Science.

84. पार्थिव द्रव्यं—Minerals (mineral substances).

85. पुरुष:—The primaeval man, as the soul and original source of the Universe; the Supreme Being, Supreme spirit.

86. प्रलय:—Dissolution of the Creation.

87. प्रतिसंस्कार—Renovation, Redoction (act of renewing).

88. प्रसाद—Essence, indispensable quality, extract.

89. प्रज्ञापराध—Intellectual blashphemy.

90. प्रकृति:—Original or primary substance, original source, nature.

91. प्रकोप:—Aggravation.

92. पुरातत्त्व—Antiquity (great age, study of archeology).

93. पुद्गल—Corporal existence of matter.

94. पूजावेतन—Scholarship for education in the Taxila University.

95. पूर्वरूप—Prodromal symptoms.

96. फल—Fruits. Vegetable product fit for food.

97. फलाशा—A temptation for the achievements.

98. बहु विवाह—Polygamy. (Practice of having more than one living consort)

99. ब्राह्मण:—A person well-versed in knowledge.

100. भेषज्य—Medicine. भेष means disease and जय means winning i.e., that which wins a disease, meaning औषधि। ओष means osmose; अधि means preservation of curative values i.e., such an osmose which preserves the curative properties.

101. भौतिकवाद—Materialism. (Tendency to attach too much importance for material things, e.g., physical comfort; money).

102. मद्य—Wines, an alchoholic drink made from grapes or other plants.

103. मनु—Mankind. The representative man and father of the human race.

104. मांस—Meat, flesh of beasts as food.

105. महान्—Intellect, faculty of knowing and reasoning, understanding.

106. मृत्युः—Death, (Death of different kinds are enumerated, mainly diseases, accidents and natural.)

107. मन्त्रः—Incantation. A formula, a gist of a matter.

108. मुनिः—A thinker on higher level.

109. यवनः—Greeks, who produced great scholars in Europe, had invaded India in 330 B.C. and continued their attacks till Alexander the Great in 326 B.C. Mostly they conquered up to Panjab. Śātavahan Kings of South India drove them away from every part of India.

110. यज्ञ यागः—Dedications for social and spiritual benefits. Sacrifices, giving something up for the sake of something else.

111. यन्त्रः—Black-art. A symbol to remove a trouble and this was taken as deified by a Siddha. A device for preparing metallic composition of medicines.

112. युगा:—A period or astronomical cycle, an age of the world, long mundane period of years of which there are four, viz., *Krita or Satya, Tretā, Dvāpara* and *Kali.*

113. यूनानि—Yavanas were titled as Yunani by Persians, while Europeans called them as Grecians. Greece remained a seat of scholars till centuries. It may not be much far off the truth that Grecians had a competitive spirit in developing knowledge with that of India.

Minender, another chieftain of Greeks, again invaded India in 150 B.C. and captured up to Shokal (Sialkot). But afterwards he was converted to Buddhism and merged with the Indian interests. Bhikṣu Nāgsen converted him to Buddhism.

Greeks developed in all the sides of knowledge—Science, Philosophy, Art, Religion, Mathematics, Astrology, and so on. Idolatry is the main concept of Greeks. Sumerians were before and were more advanced than the Greeks.

114. रजस्—The darkening quality; passion; emotion, affection. (One of the three guṇas—सत्व, रजस्, तमस्,).

115. रस:—*Rasa* is used for pure mercury in Āyurveda, which gained dominance after Nāgarjun. Six *Rasas* were chemically dominant in Āyurvedic science.

1. मधुर: 2. आम्ल: 3. लवण: 4. कटु 5. तिक्त: 6. कषाय:

Whole Pharmacopia of Āyurvedic Science depends upon these six *rasas.*

116. रसायन—A particular drug used as a vermifuge; an alchemist. (Name of various plants.)

117. रसायनी विद्या—The science of Rajuvenation, or Geriatrics. The mercurial discoveries are also said to be *'Rasayani Vidya'*. Siddhas took a dominant part in developing this science in India. Greeks also took it from them and they titled it 'Alchemy'.

Siddhas made this science a philosophy and wrote much for its supernatural achievements. Whatever it is, their discoveries proved to be a great support for the Āyurvedic System. Their attempt to convert mercury into gold could not become practicable.

118. राजधर्म—Law relating to kings, polity; state policy.

119. राष्ट्र:—A nation, having cultural, historical and geographical unity. Indians always established a 'राष्ट्र', But never a 'राज्य' because a *Rajya* is established through arms.

120. रूपम्—Appearance of a disease or symptom. This is a part of *Nidāna,* out of five parts of it.

   1. निदान, 2. पूर्वरूप, 3. रूप, 4. उपशय, 5. सम्प्राति which are called निदान पंचक।

   A patient cannot be treated unless these five points are well-known.

121. रोग:—Irregular action of *Tridoṣa.* They are,

   1. वात 2. पित्त 3. कफ

   The irregular action of these three is a disease and when they work in a regular way, health improves.

122. लंघन—Diet control as advised.

123. लोक:—Country, province, region, people.

124. लोहसिद्धि—Alchemy–A school of thought to achieve metallic compositions to obtain a stout body for enjoyment.

125. वर्णाश्रमधर्म—It is applicable to the four principal classes described in Manus' code, viz., *Brāhmaṇas; Kṣatriyas, Vaiśyas* and *Śūdras.* According to practice, duty, justice, virtue, morality, religion.

126. विचार समिति:—A cabinet to consider some serious matters.

127. विश्—The social asset of a nation.

128. विद्या—The knowledge which redeems from calamities. सा विद्या या विमुक्तये.
129. विज्ञानम्—The centrifugal thoughts are said to be ज्ञान.
130. विषमाशन—Irregular eating.
131. विक्षेप—Scattering, dispersion.
132. वेदः—The Universal knowledge. The Vedas are eternal नित्य, beginningless. अनादि and not made by man अपौरुषेय.
133. वैश्यः—Businessmen commanding national finance.
134. वैषम्य—Inequality; oddness; distress; mistake.
135. वृद्धिः—Growth; increase, come into existence; become gradually.
136. विसर्गः—Discharge; opening, rejection.
137. शाक—Vegetables.
138. शुकधान्य—Corns with bristles.
139. शाश्वतः—Eternal. Forever.
140. शिल्प—Technology. (Application of practical mechanical sciences to industry, commerce, technical methods or skills; art of forming representation by chiselling, carving etc.)
141. शिवः—Auspicious, benevolent, God Rudra.
142. श्रद्धा—Trust, Respect true faith or belief.
143. श्री—A monogram of Shiva and Gauri, denoting bliss and glory for him before it is used. (शिव + गौरी = शि+री=श्री).
144. शमीधान्यं—Pulses, throbbing in the arteries that show how fast the heart is beating. (नाडीपरीक्षा—to examine the pulse)
145. शूद्रः—One who could not be able to get education, and therefore, is bound to serve others. Still had a right to develop himself and get a better place in the society.

146. षड्रसवाद The theory of six *Rasa-viz,* मधुर, आम्ल, लवण, कटु, तिक्त, कषाय।

147. षडंग—The six attributes of the Vedas—

1. *Śikṣā,* 2. *Kalpa,* 3. *Vyākaraṇa,*
4. *Nirukta,* 5. *Chhandas,* 6. *Jyotiṣa.*

148. समशन—Mixed eating.

149. सत्व—Material or else monetary substance; matter. (as the highest of the three *Guṇas*).

150. सदाचार—Knowing the real truth; good conduct, good practice. Following with what is taught by the teacher.

151. सप्तसिन्धु—The western plateau of the Indus river containing main supplementary seven rivers :—1. Swat. 2. Kabul. 3. Kurram. 4. Gomel. 5. Zhob. 6. Nine. 7. Mari.

This country was named Gandhar with its capital named Pushkalavati. At present this place is identified by the name of Charsadda in Afghanistan.

From Hindukush to Kabul river, the land was called कपिशदेश which now is called Kafiristan. Kapish was famous for producing the best wines. Gandhar Art is famous in Indian history. Gandharvas were the masters of music. Kapish was a part of Gandhar.

After his accession Rama divided the kingdom amongst the princes of his family. He gave Taxila to the first son of Bharat named Takṣa and Pushkalavati to the second son of Bharat named Pushkal. Taxila was the capital city of Kekaya desh and Pushkalavati was that of Gandhar. Saptasindhu was a beautiful plateau of Gandhar. [vide भारत के प्राणाचार्य, by कवीराज रत्नाकर, p. 874].

152. साम्य—Normal state. Equality. षड्रस:—Six *Rasas.* मधुर—Sweet; अम्ल—Sour, लवण—salty, कटु—Pungent and तिक्त—bitter, कषाय—Astringent.

153. संस्कारा:—Making perfect; refining purification; preparation, education. A sacred rite or ceremony.

154. संयम—Control; govern; (senses; passions) To present with, give to; [*Atmane pada*—with instrumental case of person; when the action is permitted, *par*-with Dati-case—when the action is not permitted.]

155. संप्राप्ति—Pathology of a disease.

156. सूत्रम्—A thread; wire. A rule.

157. सिन्धु सभ्यता—Memories of 5000 B.C. old civilization of India, which contains a number of articles excavated from antiquity, Harappa and Mohenjodaro are the main cities where the land was excavated. The articles obtained here are very much correlated with those which are obtained in ancient Babylonia.

158. सिद्धान्त—Principle or a final decision.

159. सिद्ध तापस वर्ग—A class of Siddhas who practised Haṭhayoga. They knew much of personal magnetism.

160. सूर्य:—The Sun or its deity. In the Vedas the name Surya is generally distinguished from Savitris and denotes the most concrete of solar gods.

161. सेन्द्रिय—Organic Element. The things which contain carbon, hydrogen and oxygen mainly.

162. स्मृति:—Remembrance; thinking of or upon; calling to mind memory. मंत्रs and ब्राह्मणs are called श्रुति, while the सूत्र are called स्मृति. The श्रुति, is what is heard, as opposed to what is composed or remembered, it is a revealed scripture; self-evident and self-authoritative, not composed by any human author. Great writer Kumārila remarks—

पूर्वविज्ञानविषयं विज्ञानं स्मृतिरुच्यते।
पूर्वज्ञानाज्ञिना तस्या: प्रामाण्यं नावधीर्यते।।

163. स्वधर्म—Own duty, moral or legal obligation. Office function.

164. श्रेणी—Category, one of the divisions in a classification, one of certain general classes.

165. सोम—Juice; extract, the juice of the Soma plant, a drug of supposed magical properties.

166. हरित—Salads, green, mixed vegetables or fruits, used as food without cooking.

167. हवनः—The exchange of benefits for the society. The dedication is the main theme of this exchange.

168. हिप्पोक्रिट्स—A prominent physician of Greece who lived in C. 460-360 B.C. Hippocrates is called the 'Father of Medicine' because he first cultivated the subject as science in Europe.

169. हिन्दू—In Persian dialect 'सिन्धु' is called 'हिन्दू'. There was no Hindu before the Persian invasions against India when the western coast of Sindhu was on revolt, the eastern land was called a country of Sindhu.

170. क्षत्रिय—Persons working in defence of a nation. Gradually it became a caste in India.

171. त्रिदोष—The biophysical organic phenomena complex in Āyurveda. *Tridoṣas* are as below :—

    1. वात—Actomorphic biophysical phenomena complex.

    2. पित्त—Mexomorphic biophysical phenomena complex.

    3. कफ—Endomorphic biophysical phenomena complex.

172. ज्ञान—A knowledge through the centripetal forces of the brain.

173. ज्ञाता—The subjective of a knowledge.

174. ज्ञेय—The object of a knowledge.

SELECT BIBLIOGRAPHY

I Sanskrit

Abhilaśitāratha cintāmaṇi of Someśvara, Part I, Ed. by Śāmaśāstri R., Mysore, 1926.

Agnipurāṇa—Anandāśrama Sanskrita Granthavali. Ed. Hari Narayan Apte, Anandasrama Press, Poona, 1900.

Āyurveda Granthāvali—Carakasaṁhitā; Suśruta Saṁhita Aṣṭāṅgahṛdayam Ed. by Rajendranath Sharma. Nag Publications, Delhi, 2001.

Bṛhatsaṁhitā of Varāhamihira, Ed. by Khemaraja Srikrishnadas; Sri Venkateswara Steam Press, Bombay, 1874.

Mādhava Nidānam, (Purvārdha) Comm. by Madhukesh, Chowkhambha Sanskrit Samsthana, Varanasi, 1981.

Mahābhārata, Vols. I-IV; Bhandarkar Oriental Research Institute, Poona, 1971-1975.

Manusmṛti, Ed. by Pandit Haragovinda Śāstri, Chowkhamba Sanskrit Office, Varanasi, 1979.

Ṛgveda, Ed. by S.D. Satavalekar, Poona.

Sanskrita Kavi Jivitam, by P. Sriramachandradu and V. Sundarasarma, Sanskrit Academy, Osmania University, Hyderabad,1982.

Taittariya Saṁhita, Government Oriental Library Series, Printed at the Government Branch Press, Mysore, 1898.

Vālmīki Rāmāyaṇa—Vol.I and II. Ed. by T.R. Krishnacharya, Śri Satguru Publications, Delhi, 1982.

II. English

Agniveśa (P.I.), *Carakasaṁhitā* (with comm. of Caraka and Dṛdhabala), Choukhamba Publications, Banaras, 1937.

Bhattacharyya B., *The Science of Tridoṣa,* (IInd Edition), Gotham Book Mart, New York, 1956.

Bhishagranta, K.L., *Suśruta Saṁhita* (English Translation), Vols. I and II, Chowkhamba Sanskrit Series Office, Varanasi, 1991.

Chakraberty, Chandra, *Interpretation of Ancient Hindu medicine,* Chakraberty R. Publications, Calcutta 1923.

Dandekar, R.N., *Source of Ancient Indian Polity,* B.K. Barua Comm. Vol., Gauhati, 1966.

Desai, P.B., *Karnataka Inscription Series,* Vol. V, Karnatak University, Dharwad, 1969.

Desai P.B. [Chief Ed.] and others, *A History of Karnataka,* Kannada Research Institute, Dharwad 1981.

Iyer, Ramamurthi T.G., *The Hand Book of Indian Medicine*, Śrī Satguru Publications, Delhi, 1981.

Joshi, M.N., *The Principles of Āyurveda—A collection* (आयुर्वेदोपदेशसंग्रहः), Roopa Publications, Dharwad, 1999.

Khemaraj Śrīkṛṣṇadās, *Aṣṭāṅgahṛdaya Saṁhita of Vāgbhata,* With English Introduction, 1891, Published by Author, Bombay, 1980.

Mehta, D.D., *Positive Science in the Vedas,* Arnold Heinemann, New Delhi, 1974.

Ramachandra Iyer, *A short History of Sanskrit Literature,* T.K. Publisher. Kalpathi 1977.

Ranade and others, *Health and disease in Āyurveda and Yoga,* Anmol Publications. Pune, 1997.

Robert Svoboda and Arnie Lade, *Chinese Medicine and Āyurveda,* Motilal Banarsidass Publications Pvt. Ltd., Delhi,1998.

Sarmapriya Vrita, *Āyurvedīya Anusandhāna Paddhati,* Chaukhamba Orientalia, Varanasi,1976.

Savnur, S.V., *A Hand Book of Āyurvedic Materia Medica* Vol. I, Dr. Jathar and Sons. Maruti Street, Belgaum, 1950.

Shama Sastry, *Āyurveda Sūtram* (with comm. of Yogānanda), Oriental Library Publications, Mysore, 1992.

Sharma, P.V., *Introduction of Dravyaguṇa,* Chaukhamba Orientalia, Varanasi, 1976.

Sharma, Priyavrat, *Essentials of Āyurveda—Ṣoḍaśāngahṛdayam,* Motilal Banarasidass Publishers Pvt. Ltd., Delhi, 1998.

Sharma, R.K. and Bhagwan Dash, *Carakasaṁhitā,* Vol. I and II. Chowkhamba Sanskrit Series Office, Varanasi, 1985.

Shrigondekar, G.K., *The Mānasollāsa of King Bhūlokamalla Someśvara,* (Three Volumes). Oriental Institute, Baroda. [1st Vol. IInd Ed. 1967; Vol. II, 1939; Vol. III, 1961].

Singhal, G.D., *Ancient Indian Surgery,* Dr. G.D. Singhal Publications, Allahabad, 1972.

Sudhama Miśra Śāstri (Illus) [Ed.], *Suśruta Saṁhitā,* Chowkhambha Publications, Banaras, 1940.

Upadhaya Yadunandana (ed.),, *Vāgabhata's Aṣṭāṅghṛdayam* (with comm. by Arideva Gupta), Chowkhamba Publishers, Banaras, 1950.

Vaidya Bhagwan Dash, *Fundamentals of Āyurvedic Medicine,* Vol. III, Bansilal and Co. New Delhi, 1982.

III Hindi

प्रियव्रतशर्मा, आयुर्वेदका वैज्ञानिक इतिहास—चौखम्बा प्रकाशन, वनारस, 1985.

विद्यालंकार अत्रिदेव, आयुर्वेदका ब्रहत् इतिहास—उत्तरप्रदेशसरकार, लखनउ, 1976.

आयुर्वेदाचार्य रणजित् रॉय् देसाई, आयुर्वेदीय हितोपदेश—श्री वैद्यनाथ आयुर्वेद भवन लि०, कलकत्ता,1994.

योगेश्वर झा, आयुर्वेद विज्ञानसारः—(Ed. with notes in Hindi by Brahmasanskara Sastri) चौखम्बा प्रकाशन, बनारस, 1945.

कविराज रत्नाकर शास्त्री, भारत के प्राणाचार्य, आत्माराम एण्ड सन्स्, दिल्ली, 1977.

आयुर्वेदाचार्य भास्कर गोविन्द घाणेकर, वैद्यकीय सुभाषित साहित्यम्, चौखम्बा संस्कृत संस्थान, वनारस, 1997.

INDEX

A

B

C

D

E

F

G

H

I

J

Y

HINDI